Comprehensive Manuals of Surgical Specialties

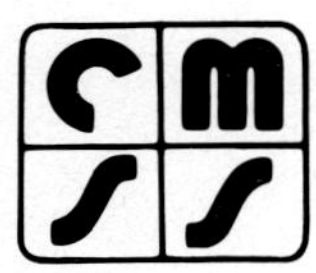

Richard H. Egdahl, editor

William H. ReMine W. Spencer Payne Jon A. van Heerden

Manual of Upper Gastrointestinal Surgery

Illustrated by Floyd E. Hosmer

Includes 139 illustrations, mostly in full color

Springer-Verlag
New York Berlin Heidelberg Tokyo

SERIES EDITOR

Richard H. Egdahl, M.D., Ph.D., Professor of Surgery, Boston University Medical Center, Boston, Massachusetts 02118, USA

William H. ReMine, M.D., M.S. (Surg.), D.Sc. (Hon.), Emeritus Professor of Surgery, Mayo Medical School; Emeritus Consultant, Section of Gastroenterologic and General Surgery, Mayo Clinic and Mayo Foundation, Rochester, Minnesota 55905, USA

W. Spencer Payne, M.D., M.S., Professor of Surgery, Mayo Medical School; Consultant, Section of Thoracic and Cardiovascular Surgery, Mayo Clinic and Mayo Foundation, Rochester, Minnesota 55905, USA

Jon A. van Heerden, M.B., Ch.B. (Cape Town), F.R.C.S. (C), Professor of Surgery, Mayo Medical School, Consultant; Section of Gastroenterologic and General Surgery, Mayo Clinic and Mayo Foundation, Rochester, Minnesota 55905, USA

Floyd E. Hosmer, M.S., A.M.I., Medical Illustrator, Section of Medical Graphics, Mayo Clinic and Mayo Foundation, Rochester, Minnesota 55905, USA

Library of Congress Cataloging-in-Publication Data
ReMine, William Hervey, 1918-
Manual of upper gastrointestinal surgery.
(Comprehensive manuals of surgical specialties)
Bibliography: p.
Includes index.
1. Esophagus—Surgery. 2. Esophagogastric junction—Surgery. 3. Peptic ulcer—Surgery. 4. Stomach—Surgery. I. Payne, W. Spencer (William Spencer), 1926- . II. Van Heerden, Jonathan A., 1938- . III. Title. IV. Series.
[DNLM: 1. Gastrointestinal System—surgery. WI 900 R388m]
RD540.R45 1985 617'.548 85-12553

Typeset by Bi-Comp, Inc., York, Pennsylvania.
Printed and bound by Universitätsdruckerei H. Stürtz AG, Würzburg/Federal Republic of Germany
Printed in the Federal Republic of Germany

9 8 7 6 5 4 3 2 1

ISBN 0-387-96148-8 Springer-Verlag New York Berlin Heidelberg Tokyo
ISBN 3-540-96148-8 Springer-Verlag Berlin Heidelberg New York Tokyo

This manual is dedicated to our many surgical colleagues at the Mayo Clinic whose vast experience in upper gastrointestinal surgery has made this book possible.

Editor's Note

Comprehensive Manuals of Surgical Specialties is a series of surgical manuals designed to present current operative techniques and to explore various aspects of diagnosis and treatment. The series features a unique format with emphasis on large, detailed, full-color illustrations, schematic charts, and photographs to demonstrate integral steps in surgical procedures.

Each manual focuses on a specific region or topic and describes surgical anatomy, physiology, pathology, diagnosis, and operative treatment. Operative techniques and stratagems for dealing with surgically correctable disorders are described in detail. Illustrations are primarily depicted from the surgeon's viewpoint to enhance clarity and comprehension.

Other volumes in the series:

Published:

Manual of Burns
Manual of Surgery of the Gallbladder, Bile Ducts, and Exocrine Pancreas
Manual of Gynecologic Surgery
Manual of Urologic Surgery
Manual of Lower Gastrointestinal Surgery
Manual of Vascular Surgery, Volume I
Manual of Cardiac Surgery, Volume I
Manual of Cardiac Surgery, Volume II
Manual of Liver Surgery
Manual of Ambulatory Surgery
Manual of Pulmonary Surgery
Manual of Soft-Tissue Tumor Surgery
Manual of Endocrine Surgery (Second Edition)
Manual of Vascular Access, Organ Donation, and Transplantation
Manual of Aesthetic Surgery

In Preparation:

Manual of Vascular Surgery, Volume II
Manual of Orthopedic Surgery

Manual of Trauma Surgery
Manual of Reconstructive Surgery
Manual of Sports Surgery
Manual of Gynecologic Surgery (Second Edition)

Richard H. Egdahl

Preface

The *Manual of Upper Gastrointestinal Surgery* was compiled as an aid to surgeons, residents, and students who want to acquire a broader knowledge of the surgical techniques used in the upper gastrointestinal area. Of necessity, a considerable amount of the work of a general surgeon will be confined to this region.

The techniques described herein are those preferred by the authors and most, but not all, of their colleagues at the Mayo Clinic. No attempt has been made to include all of the available possibilities and technical variations. Likewise, no attempt has been made to include many of the stapling techniques. Although they are good and quite useful, their inclusion would require a complete and separate volume. The omission of an accepted procedure is not meant as a criticism; our aim was to emphasize only the techniques that are most commonly used in day-to-day practice.

Gains in knowledge about the anatomy and physiology of the esophagus, stomach, and duodenum have been highly instrumental in the development of surgical procedures in these areas, particularly the techniques for benign diseases (for example, ulcer, gastritis, and esophagitis).

In the United States, operations for malignant lesions of the stomach have become infrequent because of the sharp decline in the incidence of gastric carcinoma. In 1935, the incidence was 36 per 100,000 population; currently, the incidence is 4 per 100,000 population. The reasons for this dramatic decline remain unclear, but they may quite possibly be due to the remarkable changes in food preservation and to the sharp decline in oral use of various forms of tobacco. Alternatively, the incidence of carcinoma of the esophagus has not shown a comparable decline.

William H. ReMine
W. Spencer Payne
Jon A. van Heerden

Acknowledgements

We wish to express our gratitude and deep appreciation to the many people who made this volume possible. They include our current colleagues, the administration of the Mayo Clinic for its understanding and cooperation, our families for allowing us the time, and members of the Section of Publications for their able assistance in preparing our manuscripts, especially LeAnn Stee for her editorial contribution.

We are highly appreciative of members of the Section of Medical Graphics for their patience, advice, and encouragement, especially Mr. Robert C. Benassi and Mr. Vincent P. Destro, who gave freely of their time and superb talents to advise us and support this project.

The authors are especially grateful to Mr. Floyd E. Hosmer for his dedication to producing a compilation of artwork of the highest quality and accuracy.

Contents

The Esophagus and Esophagogastric Junction

1

W. Spencer Payne

Surgical Anatomy

The esophagus is basically a hollow, squamous epithelial-lined conduit between the hypopharynx and the stomach. It extends from the cricopharyngeal muscle (upper esophageal sphincter) at the level of the sixth cervical vertebra to a point 2 cm below the diaphragm, where it joins the stomach. In the thorax, the esophagus is a vertical, tubular, posterior, mediastinal structure ensheathed by an inner layer of circular muscle and an outer layer of longitudinal muscle. Its outer aspect is in contact with the loose areolar connective tissues of the mediastinum. It totally lacks a visceral serosal covering, although the mediastinal pleura covers the right lateral aspect of almost the entire length of the thoracic esophagus. The musculature of its upper third is striated and that of the lower two-thirds is smooth. The smooth muscle in the lower 4 to 6 cm of the esophagus makes up the highly specialized lower esophageal sphincter. On gross inspection, the lower esophageal sphincter is only subtly differentiated from the rest of the esophagus. In this area there is thickening of the inner circular smooth muscle, which, in association with the longitudinal muscle, blends imperceptibly with the musculature of the stomach.

The stratified squamous epithelial lining of the esophagus is continuous above with that of the oral and pharyngeal mucosa. Distally, this lining abruptly ends at a discrete squamocolumnar epithelial line at the esophagogastric junction. Because this junctional transition line is not a straight horizontal line but is often zigzag, it is often referred to as the "Z line." About a third of normal persons will have at least one island or patch of columnar epithelium from 1 to 30 mm in diameter located at random points throughout an otherwise squamous, epithelial-lined esophagus. Most of these developmental epithelial rests occur high in the thoracic esophagus and are commonly a ciliated respiratory type of epithelium, although gastric epithelium has been described. In the submucosa throughout the length of the esophagus are scattered microscopic mucous glands that secrete into the esophageal lumen.

The esophagus develops specific spatial relationships with various organs and structures as it descends through the thorax (Fig. 1-1). It rests on thoracic vertebral bodies throughout most of its course. As it enters the chest from above, it is a midline structure directly behind the membranous

Figure 1-1

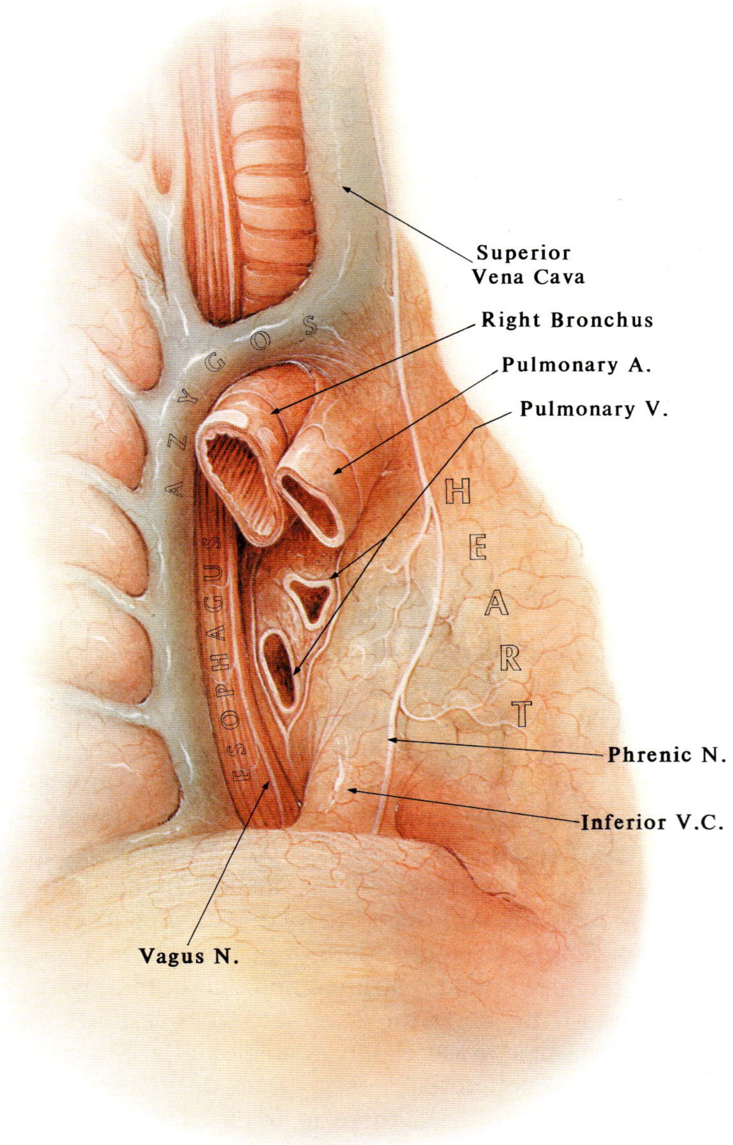

aspect of the trachea. It deviates slightly to the left of the midline as it descends to pass behind the left main-stem bronchus and the left atrium. Higher, it is indented on its left by the arch of the aorta; on the right, it is crossed by the azygos vein at the level the vein joins the superior vena cava. From the level of the arch of the aorta distally, the esophagus parallels the descending thoracic aorta, which lies to its left, until both structures penetrate their respective diaphragmatic hiatuses to enter the abdomen. Several centimeters above the diaphragm, the esophagus deviates to the left behind the pericardial sac and passes through the esophageal hiatus in front of the aorta and its hiatus. In these lower few centimeters, the esophagus briefly loses its proximity with the right pleural space and comes in contact with the mediastinal pleura of the left pleural space and the left inferior pulmonary ligament. The thoracic duct enters the thorax from below through the aortic hiatus of the diaphragm but lies posteriorly between the esophagus and aorta throughout its course to the

Figure 1-2

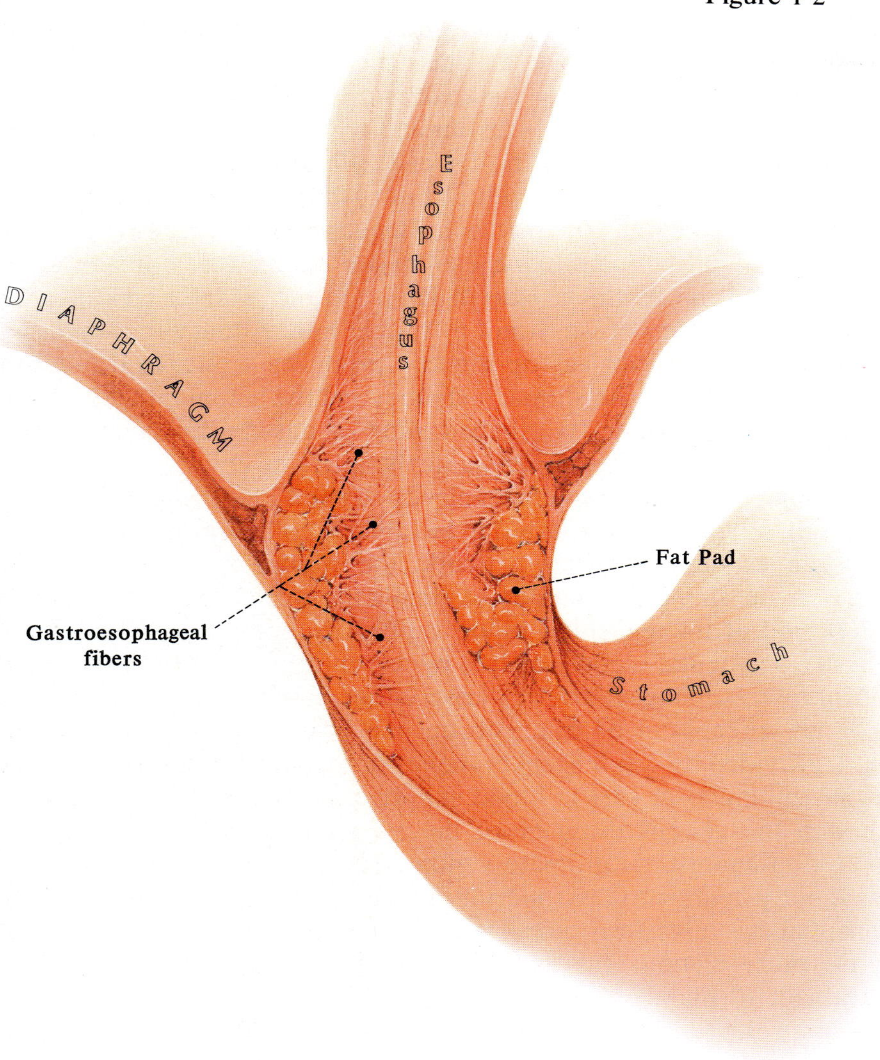

level of the aortic arch, where the duct deviates away from the esophagus to follow the left subclavian vessels to the neck.

The relationship of the esophagus to the stomach and the supporting structures of the diaphragm is important to the subsequent discussion of gastroesophageal function.

Both the esophageal and the aortic hiatus are more than simple fenestrations in the diaphragm. Both tubular structures pass through definable loops of diaphragmatic musculature called crura. Although the crura have some variation in their precise anatomic arrangement, they consistently arise from the lateral aspects of the second, third, and fourth lumbar vertebral bodies and ascend to loop about the esophageal hiatus.

Within the esophageal hiatus of the diaphragm are supporting attachments that anchor the esophagus to the undersurface of the diaphragm. The most important of these attachments is the phrenoesophageal ligament or membrane. This structure is basically a continuation of transversalis fascia along the undersurface of the diaphragm; it inserts onto the circumference of the esophagus and prevents cephalad displacement of the lower part of the esophagus. Because the fibers of the phrenoesophageal ligament insert into a fairly wide collar of distal esophagus, the interstices of its fibers are filled and surrounded with loose, fatty areolar connective tissue (the esophagogastric fat pad) (Fig. 1-2).

Normally, there is approximately 2 cm of intra-abdominal esophagus before the esophagus joins the stomach. Because of the eccentric globular configuration of the stomach, the esophagus enters the stomach at an acute angle with the fundus (angle of His). On the lesser curvature, the angle of entry is more obtuse, if not a straight line. About the esophageal introitus, loose redundant gastric mucosa produces a puckered mucosal plug. Within the wall of the stomach just beyond the actual introitus of the esophagus is an intramural U-shaped sling of gastric musculature that loops around the esophageal opening at the angle of His.

The esophagus receives a rich segmental arterial blood supply throughout its length but also maintains a rich intramural collateral arterial circulation. As a consequence of this network, the inferior thyroid vessels are capable of maintaining the viability of almost the entire length of an esophagus deprived of its segmental blood supply. Nonetheless, there is normally a rich segmental blood supply downward from the level of the aortic arch. Multiple esophageal arteries arise either directly from the adjacent aorta or via intercostal or tracheobronchial branches. Additional blood supply is provided by esophageal branches of the inferior phrenic arteries, and a rich submucosal gastric blood supply is provided from below.

Although the venous drainage of the esophagus tends to parallel the arterial blood supply, its ultimate venous drainage is via the azygos and hemiazygos systems into the superior vena cava. Small, submucosal, vertical esophageal veins form important collateral venous connections between the portal venous circulation of the stomach and the systemic venous drainage of the esophagus.

Lymphatic channels run longitudinally in the wall of the esophagus throughout its length. These channels drain via penetrating channels to reach periesophageal lymph nodes in the neck, mediastinum, and subdiaphragmatic, gastric, celiac, and periaortic nodal areas.

Although the esophagus is richly innervated by both sympathetic and parasympathetic fibers, only parasympathetic innervation is of surgical interest. This innervation is provided exclusively by the vagi. The recurrent laryngeal nerves provide, in addition to vocal cord function, an important nerve supply to the upper esophageal sphincter and upper third of the esophagus. The main trunks of the vagi lie on either side of the esophagus through most of its upper course; they form a variable plexus about the esophagus in its middle third and finally reunite as anterior and posterior vagal trunks that pass through the esophageal hiatus onto the stomach and the remainder of the digestive tract.

Physiology

The function of the esophagus is largely that of a nonabsorbing dynamic conduit for the transport of oral secretions and ingested nutrients to the stomach. As a descriptive physiologic event, swallowing begins in the mouth and terminates at the esophagogastric junction. Although the sequential oral, pharyngeal, and esophageal phases of swallowing are definable and each is essential to a safe and effective mechanism, only the esophageal phase is relative to this text.

The conduction of solids and liquids down the esophagus is aided by both gravity and motor propulsion. The latter is a highly complex, sequential neuromuscular event coordinated in the brainstem with the oral and pharyngeal phases of swallowing. The actual esophageal events are quite simple, however: sequential, peristaltic muscular contraction from top to bottom.

The esophagogastric junction plays a special role in these coordinated events; superimposed on the basic propulsive conduit function of the esophagus is a widely appreciated, but poorly understood, competence mechanism (Fig. 1-3). Simply stated, this physiologic mechanism retards the retrograde flow of reservoir (stomach) contents into the conduit (esophagus).

The need for a competence mechanism is compelling, but potent forces frustrate it. The injurious effects of refluxed upper digestive secretions on the esophageal mucosa and lung (if respiratory aspiration occurs) constitute the major need for the competence mechanism.

The main forces in conflict with competence at the cardia relate to the ambient pressures of body cavities traversed by the esophagus. Thus, the esophagus passes from the negative intrathoracic pressure of the chest to a positive intra-abdominal pressure. As a result, existing resting and dynamic pressure gradients per se are conducive to retrograde flow or reflux.

The major mechanisms antagonistic to reflux are (1) the resting tone of the intrinsic smooth muscle sphincter of the lower esophagus and (2) the augmentation of that tone in the short segment of intra-abdominal esophagus exposed to the positive pressures of the abdomen. These two mechanisms are believed to be responsible for the generation of a high-pressure zone in the distal esophagus of normal persons that provides an intraluminal pressure barrier to gastroesophageal reflux. Ancillary factors, such as the esophageal crura, the phrenoesophageal ligament, the oblique muscular sling fibers of the stomach, the gastric mucosal rosette, the oblique angle of esophageal entry, and the flap valve effected by an acute angle of His, are largely supportive or passive contributors to competence. Undoubtedly, certain digestive hormones and secretions, foodstuffs, chemicals, and drugs can have a profound modifying effect on the resting tone and function of the lower esophageal sphincter, but basic coordination with the act of swallowing is exclusively a neuromuscular event mediated through vagi. Thus, on swallowing, the lower esophageal sphincter almost immediately relaxes in anticipation of the arrival of a bolus and the subsequent peristaltic wave. Sphincteric contraction occurs as the peristaltic wave passes through the sphincter. After contraction, the lower esophageal sphincter relaxes to its resting but elevated tone. One of the salient features of this sphincter is that its resting tone responds to an increase in intragastric pressure by an equivalent rise in its own pressure. This reflex mechanism further prevents reflux of gastric contents and is an important aspect of competence.

Other protective mechanisms include the presence of an upper esophageal sphincter for the prevention of respiratory aspiration. The tone of the upper sphincter is linked with changes in intrathoracic pressure, presumably to prevent esophageal breathing. Its tone is also increased with retrograde distention of the lower esophagus.

Obviously, the viscosity, volume, and composition of saliva are important for diluting, coating, lubricating, buffering, and protecting the esopha-

Figure 1-3 A

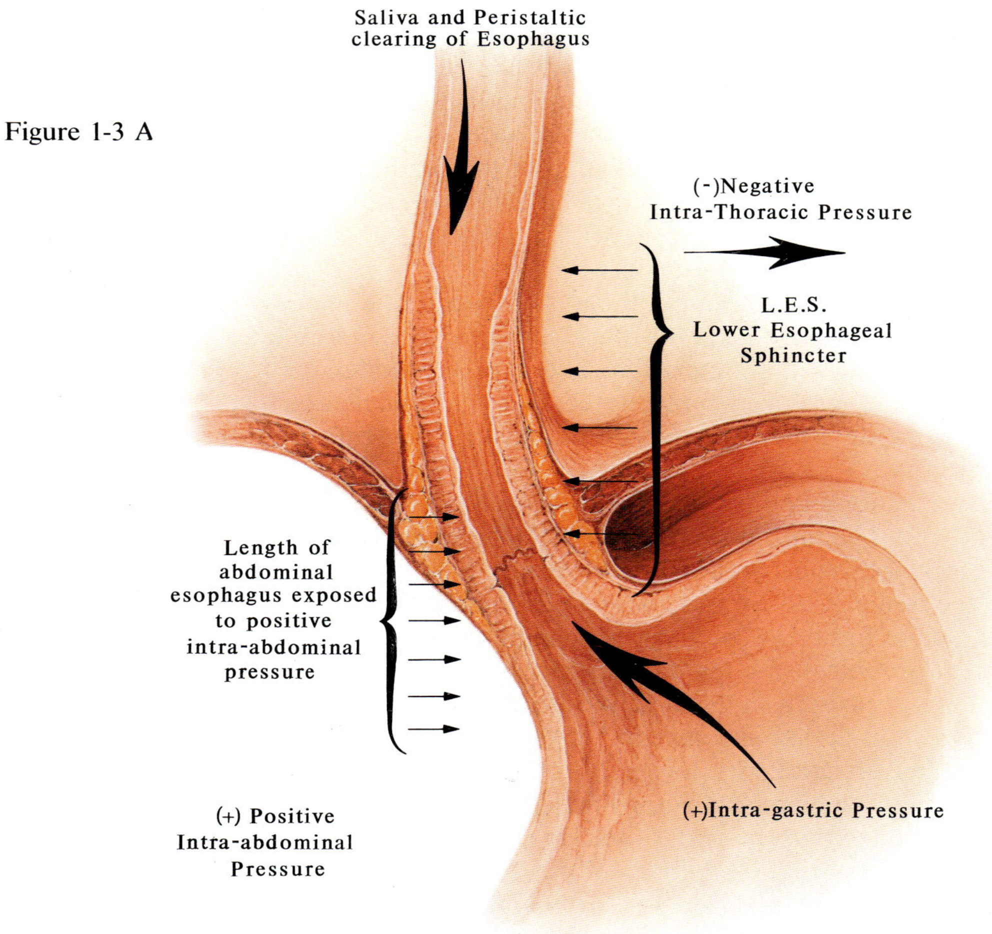

geal mucosa. More than a liter of this fluid is formed and swallowed daily, largely as an insensible activity.

With either voluntary or insensible swallowing, primary peristalsis clears refluxed material from the esophagus from top to bottom. In addition, the lower esophagus responds to local distention by producing a secondary peristaltic response. This important clearing mechanism also tends to keep the esophagus empty of refluxed or residual material. Various clinical procedures are used to test these and related functions, which are often altered in the presence of chronic gastroesophageal reflux. These procedures include acid-barium ingestion, acid perfusion, acid clearance, the standard acid-reflux, and, more recently, the 8- and 24-hour acid-reflux tests. Esophageal motility studies performed with multiple, simultaneous manometric recordings at three or more levels in the esophagus provide excellent information regarding primary peristalsis and the contraction and relaxation of the esophageal sphincter. Resting pressure characteristics of the lower esophageal sphincter are best defined by drawing a pressure probe through the resting lower esophagus to define its length and magnitude.

Of equal importance to reflux and its complications are events in the stomach. Obviously, intragastric pressure, the state of gastric distention, and the volume and composition of gastric contents are critical. These conditions, in turn, are dependent on gastric events and events down-

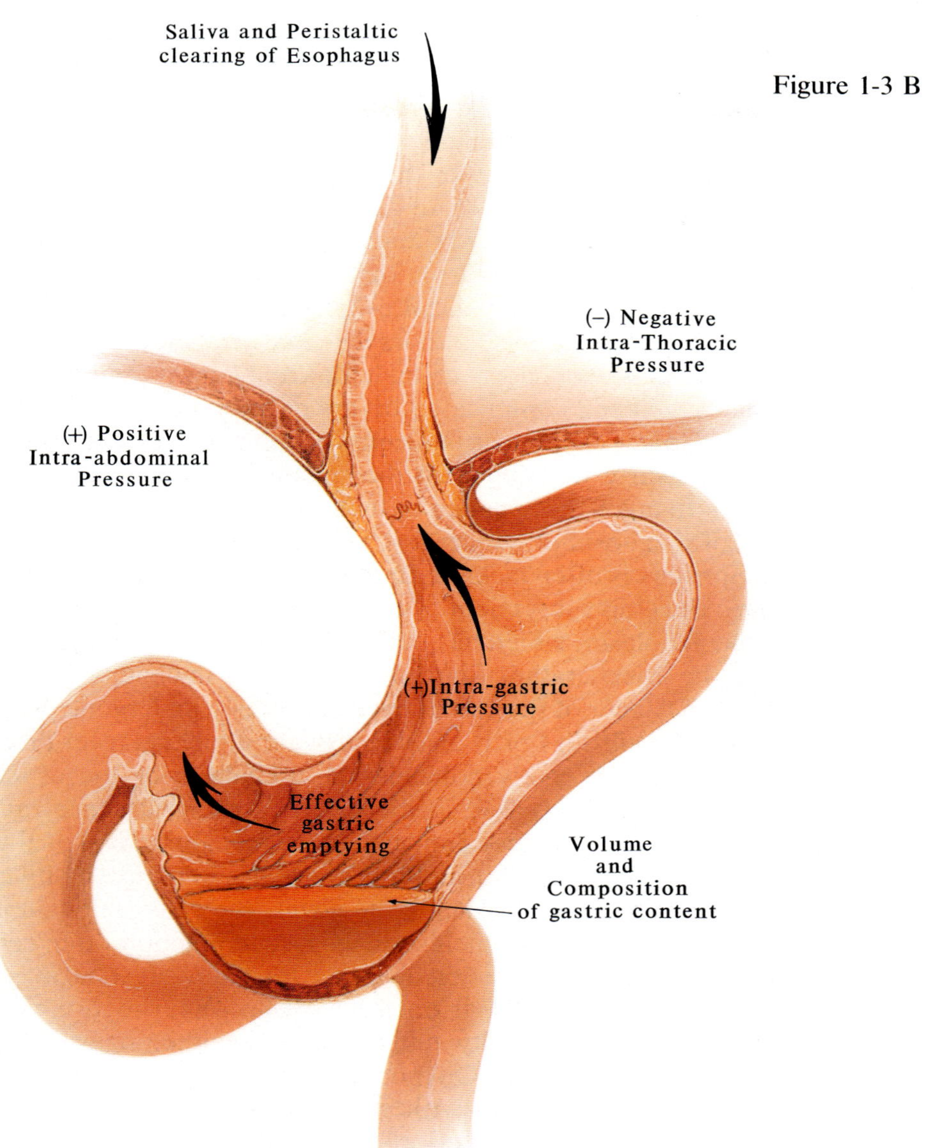

Figure 1-3 B

stream in the intestinal tract. Intragastric pressure is dependent on intra-abdominal pressure as well as on the state of gastric distention with food and secretions. Gastric emptying also is a factor in reflux; it is indirectly related to the patency of the distal gastrointestinal tract and to gastric innervation, tone, and motility.

The exquisite sensitivity of the esophageal mucosa to upper digestive secretions is responsible for the esophageal complication of gastroesophageal reflux. Even though acid-peptic secretions have been correctly implicated, it is increasingly apparent that biliary-pancreatic secretions can be equally corrosive. Thus, even in the presence of achlorhydria or a total gastrectomy, significant reflux esophagitis can occur if these secretions can gain access to the lining of the esophagus. Obviously, mixed acid-peptic and biliary-pancreatic reflux esophagitis can occur after pyloroplasty or gastroenterostomy. In the presence of incompetence at the cardia, the type and concentration of digestive secretions and mucosal resistance, as well as total contact time with the esophagus, influence the severity of injury.

Carcinoma of the Esophagogastric Junction

Approximately half of the cancers that affect the esophagus arise in the region of the esophagogastric junction. Unlike the almost ubiquitous squamous cell cancers that occur in the more proximal thoracic and cervical esophagus, approximately 90% of cancers in the cardia are adenocarcinomas and, as such, are not true primary esophageal malignant lesions. They are proximal stomach neoplasms that arise from gastric epithelium and secondarily extend onto the distal esophagus.

The precise cause of these tumors is unknown. A few have been associated with a sliding esophageal hiatal hernia and long-standing reflux esophagitis that have been complicated by the development of a columnar epithelial-lined lower esophagus (Barrett's esophagus). In some patients, the cancer has clearly developed in the region of such acquired abnormal epithelium. In many other patients, such a diaphragmatic hernia is found at the time of diagnosis of cancer but evidence for previous reflux or Barrett's esophagus is often lacking. In most instances, the anatomic hernia is thought to develop subsequent to the tumor as a result of cicatricial reaction to the neoplasm, which has pulled the esophagogastric junction cephalad into the chest, rather than to precede the malignant lesion. A few patients with cancer of the cardia have previously undergone distal gastric resection with Billroth I or II anastomosis for duodenal ulcer disease; this relationship, too, is likely coincidental. Achalasia of the esophagus is associated with an increased incidence of esophageal cancer at all anatomic levels; a few of these cancers are adenocarcinomas of the cardia. The high incidence of alcohol and tobacco abuse in patients with cancer of the cardia is impressive; basically, however, the causes remain obscure.

Clinically, neoplasms in the esophagogastric junction often remain occult until esophageal obstruction occurs. Classically, dysphagia is progressive: initially, only solid foods obstruct swallowing; progressively, softer and finer foods cause difficulty; and ultimately, neither ingested liquids nor endogenous saliva will pass. Odynophagia (painful swallowing) at the level of the neoplasm is common with cancer of the cardia. The pain in the epigastrium may radiate posteriorly to the thoracic spine or around the costal arch. Odynophagia has no prognostic significance, although it does suggest the presence of a malignant lesion. Occasionally, the neoplasm will be detected prior to any localizing symptom when diagnostic studies are initiated for occult blood-loss anemia or active upper gastrointestinal bleeding. Malignant disease at the cardia is a great masquerader of other esophageal conditions. It may mimic achalasia radiographically and on motility study; thus, irrespective of radiographic findings, all patients with dysphagia need early endoscopic examination with appropriate cytologic study and tissue biopsy.

In some patients, cancer of the cardia may manifest initially as a seemingly benign ulcer at the esophagogastric junction or in the proximal stomach. In other patients, the disease seems to have developed subtly in an area of previous chronic stricture. Finally, in a few patients with dysphagia with or without pain, cancer is clinically impossible to diagnose, with the exception of surgical exploration for open biopsy or, indeed, examination of the resected obstructing portion of the esophagus and stomach. Thus, although a definite preoperative diagnosis of malignant disease is highly desirable, resection for both diagnosis and treatment is sometimes not only justified but also desirable.

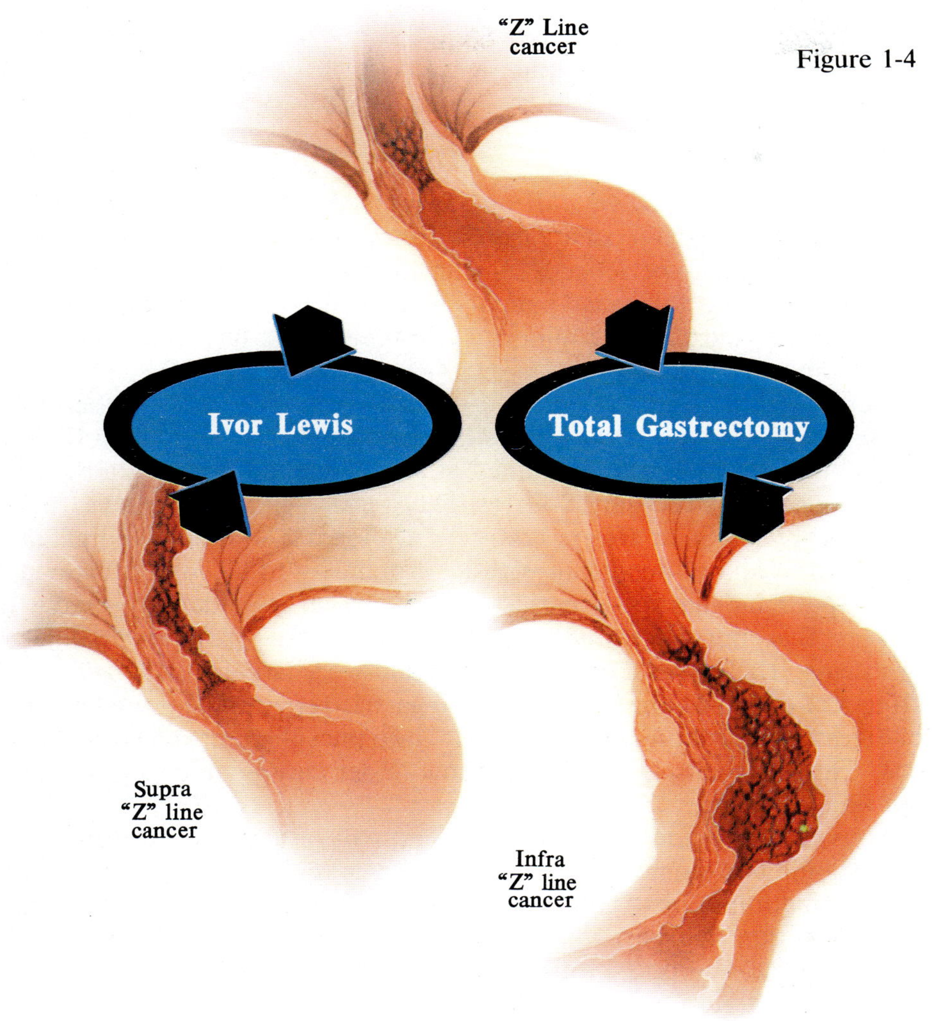

Figure 1-4

Surgical Strategies

Most patients who undergo operation for cancer of the cardia have not only a tissue diagnosis of malignant disease but also sufficient radiographic and endoscopic information to define clearly its local anatomic extent. In operable patients, treatment strategy can be planned largely on the basis of such preliminary information. The three common anatomic types of neoplastic involvement are (1) cancers that minimally involve the stomach but largely reside in the distal third of the esophagus (supra Z-line cancers), (2) cancers that seem to reside only at the esophagogastric junction with minimal extension onto either the esophagus or the stomach (Z-line cancers), and (3) cancers that are largely gastric with minimal esophageal involvement (infra Z-line cancers) (Fig. 1-4). A fourth type of neoplasm, extensive involvement of both the distal esophagus and the proximal stomach, is theoretically possible; however, experience suggests that such large neoplasms are rarely operable and, when resectable, require total esophagogastrectomy with colonic reconstruction. The anatomic extent of the neoplasm in relation to the Z line may be used to select an appropriate resection and reconstruction for common cancers of the cardia (Fig. 1-4). Two basic surgical techniques, the Ivor-Lewis esophagogastrectomy and total gastrectomy with distal esophagectomy, and the method of reconstruction will be described in detail.

Selection of Operation and Patients

A Philosophical Prologue. If one accepts the thesis that cancers of the cardia are rarely diagnosed early and that only 20% of patients who undergo resection experience a 5-year survival, then surgical efforts are clearly palliative for most patients. However, resection should not be prejudicial to cure for the minority of patients who have the potential for long-term benefit.

The most pressing subjective and objective disability of patients who present with cancer of the cardia is esophageal obstruction. In the past, surgical efforts were clearly aimed at an expedient left transthoracic partial esophagogastrectomy with esophagogastrostomy to relieve the primary problem. Such efforts restored swallowing and also eliminated the ulcerating primary neoplasm with its propensity to bleed. Unfortunately, many patients managed in this way incurred secondary digestive distresses that not infrequently overshadowed the presenting subjective problems. These late sequelae of resection were largely attributable to the effects of concomitant vagotomy with gastric retention and the free reflux of digestive secretions, especially bile, into the sphincter-deprived esophagus. Clearly, such patients had "come under care unable to swallow and left unable to eat."

Thus, the operation selected for treatment of cancer of the cardia not only should be commensurate with total removal of all gross neoplasm and the elimination of obstruction to swallowing but also should incorporate a reconstruction that permits comfortable digestion throughout subsequent survival. The two operations to be described—the Ivor-Lewis resection and total gastrectomy (Roux-Y)—have these basic attributes.

A patient selected for operation should be free of obvious distant metastatic disease. Thus, patients with skeletal, central nervous system, or cervical lymph nodal metastatic lesions are not surgical candidates, nor are patients with malignant ascites or malignant rectal shelf or pulmonary metastatic lesions. Computed tomography has been of limited value in the determination of resectability. Unless grossly palpable and biopsy proven, liver defects that are detected with any of the current methods usually do not militate against exploration. The reasons are simple. If operation cannot encompass all neoplasms, some type of surgical palliation for dysphagia should be considered.

Thus, extensive, expensive, and often nondefinitive investigations for occult metastasis have no advantage when definitive decisions can be readily made and effected at the time of exploration. Thus, whether a patient is supine in preparation for the initial stage of an Ivor-Lewis resection or positioned for a left thoracoabdominal exploration for total gastrectomy, the initial incision is always a short, limited abdominal incision that permits biopsy and pertinent exploration of the abdomen.

Generally, patients with extensive hepatic metastatic disease are excluded from resection because they have a median survival of 2.5 months. Certainly the age and general health of a patient, the mobility of a neoplasm, and active neoplastic hemorrhage influence the decision to proceed with noncurative resection if this procedure is otherwise technically feasible. Most patients with malignant disease of the cardia who are not candidates for resection have sufficient circumferential (annular) esophageal involvement that a palliative indwelling tube can be impacted into the esophagus. This conduit through the area of obstructing neoplasm gives satisfactory palliation for dysphagia during subsequent limited survival. In some patients, neoplasms that are largely gastric (infra Z-line) are not suitable for insertion of a palliative tube. In fact, the lack of esophageal involvement precludes the impaction and proper anchorage of such tubes. In such circumstances, the decision regarding whether gastrostomy or jejunostomy should be performed is largely one of expediency. Such a procedure does not prolong survival and provides no palliation for dysphagia or even the elimination of salivary secretions. However, it may provide an alternative to intravenous feeding and permit patients to become relatively independent of hospital and professional care, thus allowing them to return home for their remaining survival.

Modified Ivor-Lewis Esophagogastrectomy

Technique. The Ivor-Lewis resection and reconstruction is chiefly used for the management of Z-line and supra Z-line cancers of the lower esophagus and cardia. Chronologically, it entails an initial transabdominal phase of assessment of the neoplasm and gastric mobilization followed by a right transthoracic resection of the distal esophagus and proximal stomach in continuity. Figure 1-5 A illustrates the essential features of the resection (dark-shaded area), in which the esophagus is transected above the carinal area approximately at the level of the azygos vein and the proximal third of the stomach and high lymph nodal tissues of the lesser curvature are removed. A pyloroplasty is indicated to ensure gastric emptying after obligatory vagotomy with esophagogastric resection. Figure 1-5 B illustrates the essential features of reconstruction, wherein the tailored proximal stomach is drawn cephalad through the esophageal hiatus to the level of the azygos vein for anastomosis.

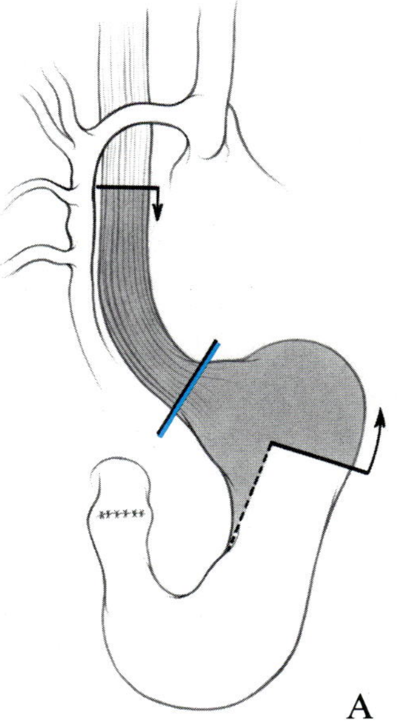

A

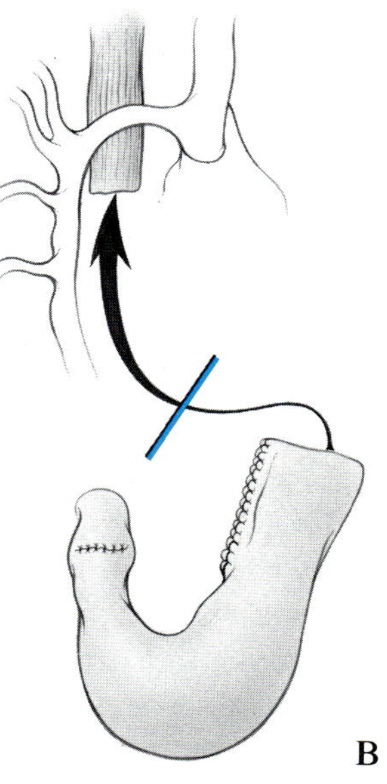

B

Figure 1-5

The sequential steps of the abdominal phase of the Ivor-Lewis procedure are shown in Figure 1-6. This phase is reliably effected with the patient in the supine position and under general anesthesia. The abdomen is explored through an upper midline incision. Exposure of the left upper quadrant is facilitated if this incision is extended cephalad into the paraxiphoid area. With retraction of the left costal arch and with the surgeon standing on the patient's right, the diaphragm and structures of the left upper quadrant are clearly viewed.

Step 1 entails sharp division of the triangular ligament to the lateral segment of the left lobe of the liver such that this segment can be retracted medially (to the right); this step permits the gastrohepatic omentum and esophagogastric junction to come into full view.

Step 2 comprises clamping, division, and ligation of the upper gastrohepatic omentum (see Fig. 1-26). The lower portion of the omentum is attenuated and avascular and can be simply divided without ligation (see Fig. 1-25).

Step 3 constitutes encirclement of the distal esophagus and vagi with transhiatal exploration and mobilization of the distal esophagus. This procedure is effected by manual downward traction of the stomach, which irons out the peritoneum over the esophagogastric junction where it reflects off the diaphragm onto the stomach. With the parietal peritoneum under tension, a horizontal incision is made to expose the anterior aspect

Figure 1-6

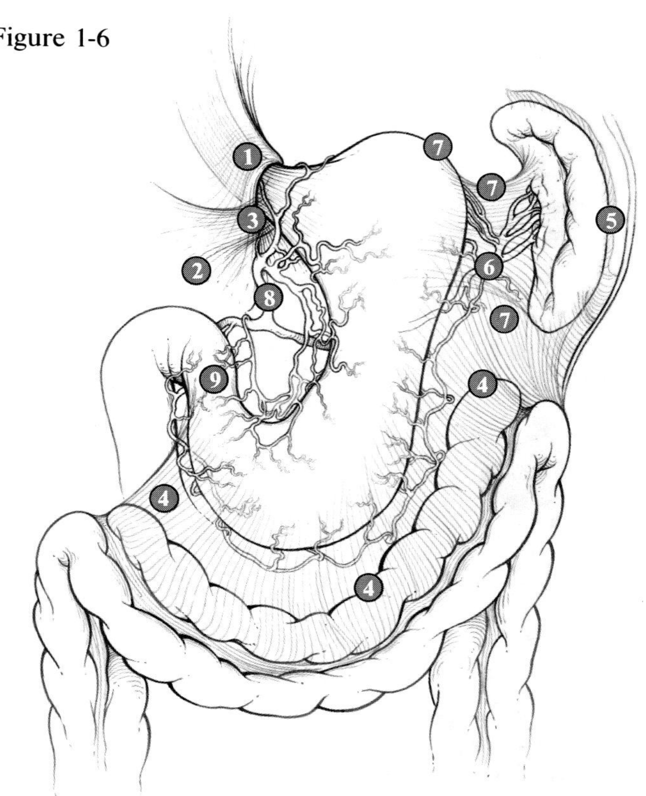

of the abdominal esophagus and vagi. By blunt digital dissection, these structures are encircled with a Penrose drain. With use of this soft rubber sling for caudad traction, the esophageal hiatus is stretched and the esophagus is bluntly mobilized by finger dissection to define the mobility of the neoplasm within the mediastinum. Specifically, one wishes to determine the freedom of the primary tumor from fixation to the aorta, vertebral bodies, or the posterior aspect of the pericardium or to determine other attachments or extensions that might technically preclude resection.

Step 4 is the beginning of gastric mobilization on the distal gastric vascular pedicles. The gastrocolic omentum is divided outside the gastroepiploic arcade from the level of the pylorus to the splenic flexure. Care is taken to preserve the right gastroepiploic blood supply to the stomach from its origin at the gastroduodenal artery on the right to the short gastric vessels on the left.

Step 5, splenectomy, is routinely effected for gastric malignant lesions of the distal esophagus. The Balfour technique of splenectomy with initial control of splenic vessels at the splenic hilus is favored. This technique entails incision of the parietal peritoneum lateral to the splenic hilus (see Fig. 1-19). This step, combined with the previous takedown of the gastrocolic omentum, permits Step 6, in which the splenic hilus is encircled with the hand (see Fig. 1-20) and the splenic vessels just distal to the tail of the pancreas are subsequently divided and doubly ligated (see Fig. 1-21 and 1-22). The spleen, thus disconnected from its hilar vessels, remains attached to the greater curvature of the stomach by short gastric vessels.

Step 7, division of the short gastric vessels to complete the splenectomy, is carried cephalad along the greater curvature of the stomach; the gastric fundus is freed by ligating all vessels and attachments of the stomach to the undersurface of the diaphragm. Because the greater and lesser curvatures of the stomach are thus completely freed of all parietal attachments from the pylorus to the esophagogastric junction, the sole remaining

Figure 1-7

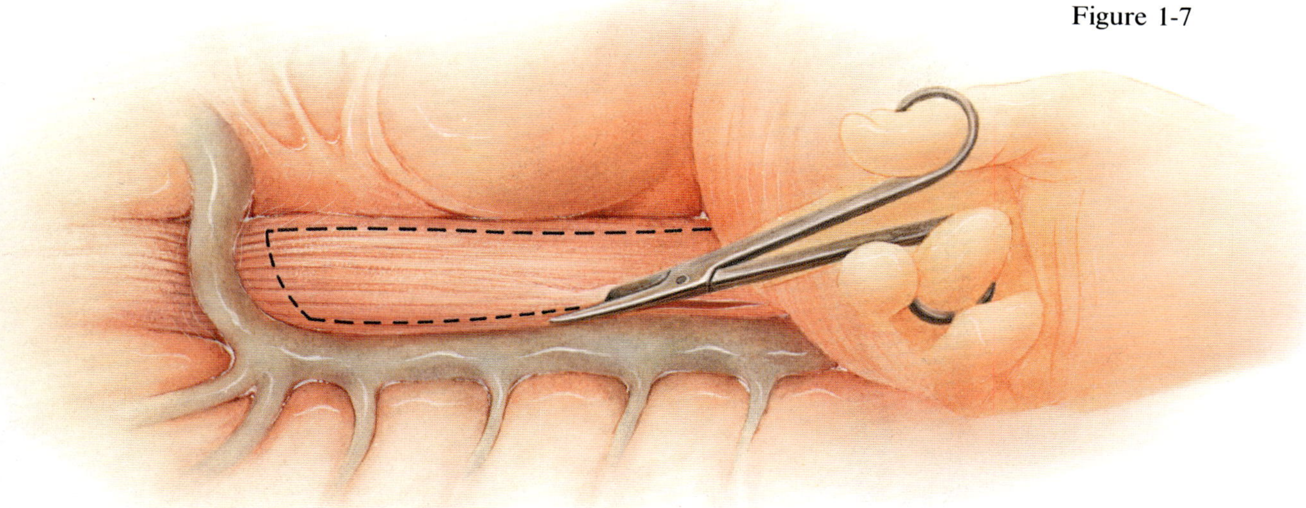

attachment, the left gastric vessels, can now be isolated, divided, and ligated (Step 8). These vessels are usually best exposed by elevating the greater curvature of the stomach to the right and isolating them behind the stomach (see Fig. 1-27). Finally, complete mobilization of the stomach from the cardia to the pylorus is ensured by passing the previously placed, esophageal-encircling Penrose drain from above distally. This maneuver ensures that the stomach can be freely brought into the chest during the second stage of the operation. The final procedure prior to abdominal closure is pyloroplasty in preparation for obligatory vagotomy. Step 9, then, is the performance of a Heineke-Mikulicz pyloroplasty using the Weinberg modification (see Fig. 3-24, 3-31, and 3-32).

After closure of the abdominal incision, the patient is placed in the left lateral decubitus position; after preparation of the right side of the chest, a midthoracic incision is made and the pleural space is entered through the periosteal bed of the nonresected right sixth rib (fifth interspace).

The use of an anesthetic tube with divided airway facilitates retraction of the right lung anteriorly to expose the esophagus (Fig. 1-7). As shown, parallel mediastinal pleural incisions are made over the lower thoracic esophagus, and a strip of mediastinal pleura is left attached to the esophagus from the diaphragm to the azygos vein. Usually, interruption of the azygos vein to gain 4 cm of tumor-free esophageal margin above the neoplasm is unnecessary. Previous transhiatal mobilization of the distal esophagus will have been accomplished during the early steps of the abdominal stage of this operation. After the pleural incisions are completed, the distal esophagus can be encircled with a Penrose drain, which provides a convenient handle for elevating the esophagus from its mediastinal bed and allows mobilization of periesophageal and subcarinal lymph nodes with the surgical specimen. Thus, the esophagus and adjacent lymph node-bearing connective tissues are mobilized from the posterior mediastinum from below upward. This maneuver should skeletonize the left pulmonary veins, left atrium, carina, both main-stem bronchi, the vertebral bodies, and the right medial aspect of the descending thoracic aorta. Electrocoagulation controls most bleeding vessels, although esophageal branches from the aorta may require ligation with fine silk suture for control.

Figure 1-8

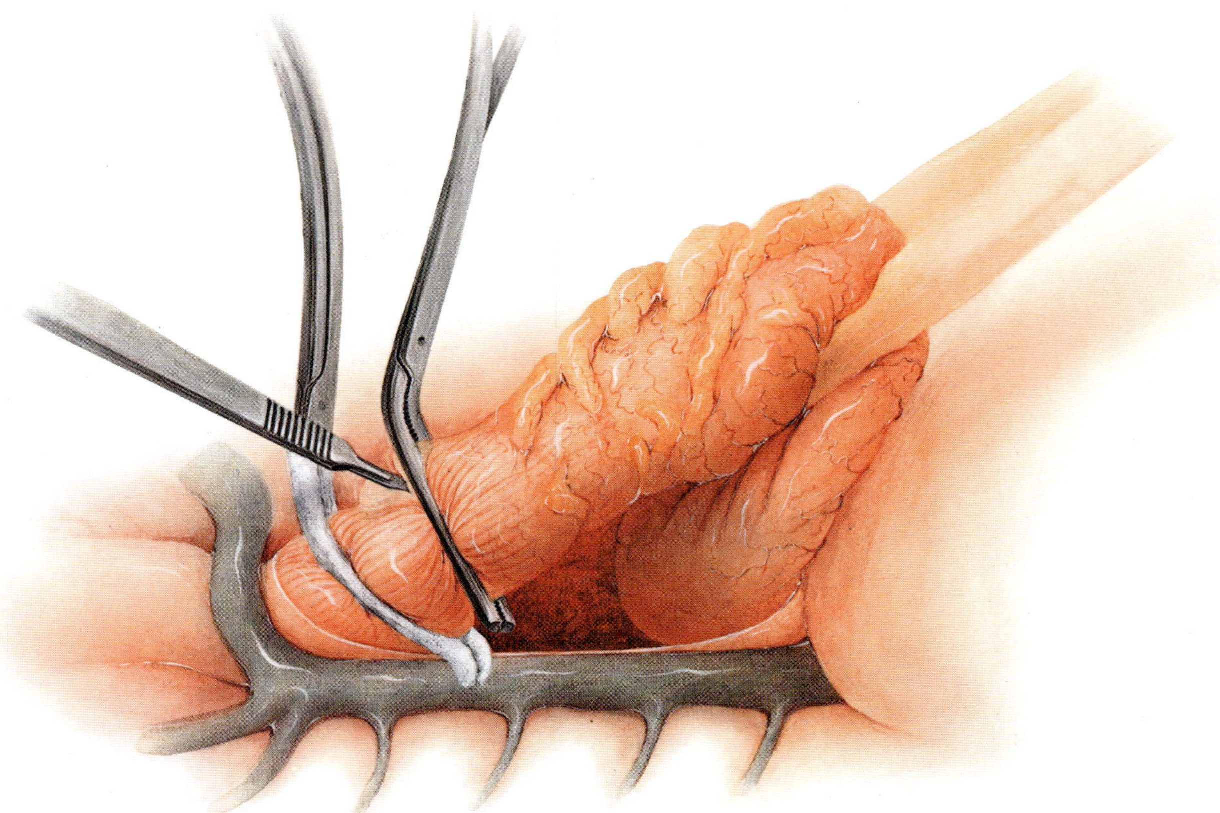

The esophagus is then transected just below the azygos vein (Fig. 1-8). Illustrated is a noncrushing, soft-fabric-shod Foss clamp applied to the upper esophagus with a scalpel used to divide the esophagus flush with a right-angled Pemberton clamp. Note that traction on the Penrose drain is beginning to draw the stomach into the chest through the esophageal hiatus.

After division of the esophagus well above the gross neoplasm, the stomach is drawn into the right side of the chest from the abdomen. With Pemberton clamps on the point of esophageal division and with the fundus of the stomach held by hand (Fig. 1-9), the vessels of the lesser curvature just distal to the left gastric ligature are clamped in preparation for division and ligation. Next, parallel curved clamps are placed at right angles to the greater curvature of the stomach at the point of gastric transection (Fig. 1-10), which should be at least 4 cm from the gross tumor. Note that the division and ligation of the vessels of the lesser curvature distal to the left gastric tie produce a clearly denuded surface for the subsequent application of a stapling device to tailor the lesser curvature. A scalpel is used to divide the stomach between the curved clamps. When this division is completed, assistants hold these clamps at right angles to one another with the tips of the clamps forming the angle (Fig. 1-11). Note that a TA 90 stapling device is applied to tailor the lesser curvature of the stomach. After delivery of staples, the esophagogastric surgical specimen is cut free of the stapling device, and curved clamps are placed on the specimen side to prevent the spillage of contents as it is cut free (Fig. 1-12).

With the original curved clamp placed on the greater curvature of the stomach at the point where the stomach will be anastomosed end-to-end with the esophagus, the lesser curvature line of staples is buried beneath a

Figure 1-9

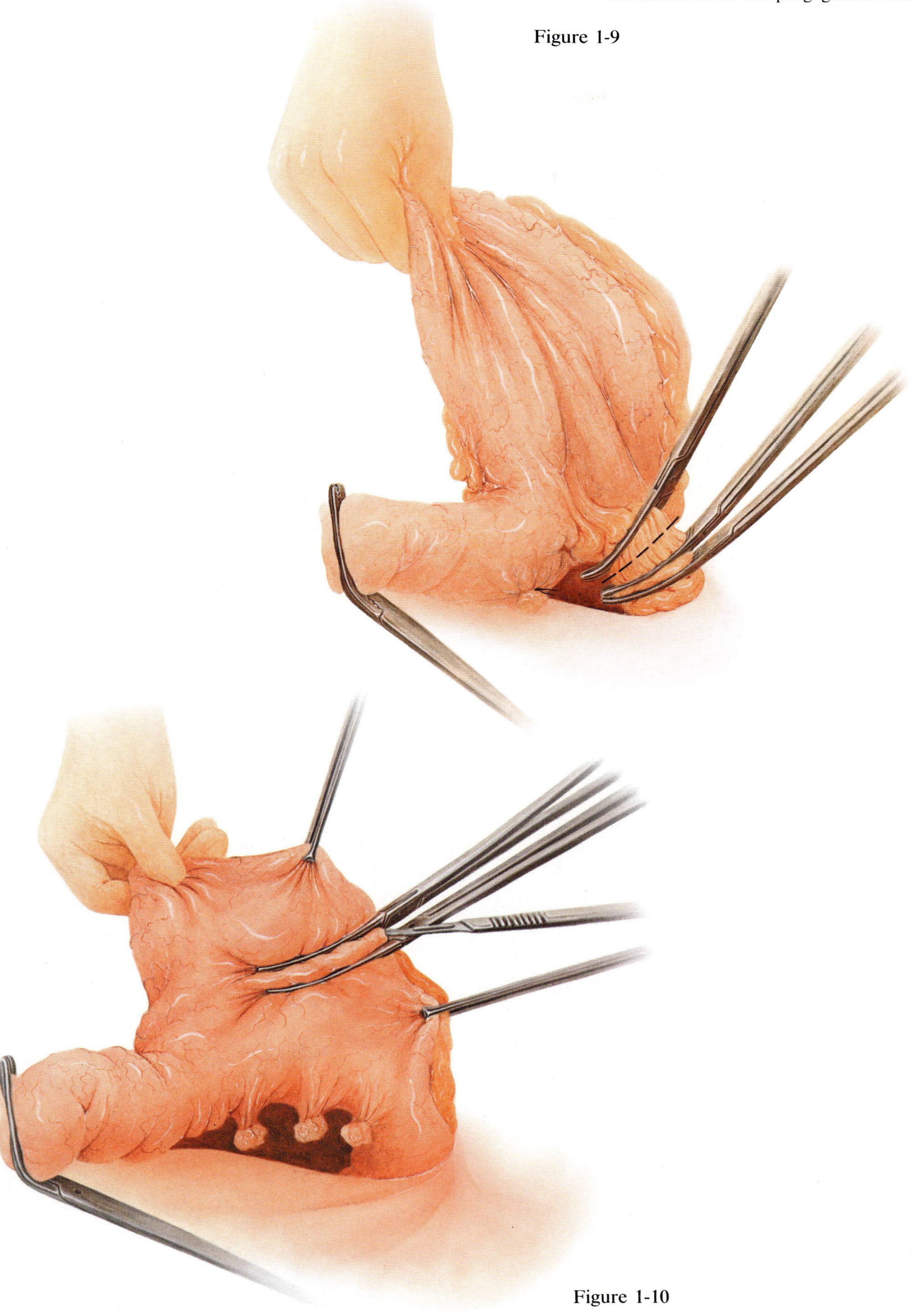

Figure 1-10

Figure 1-11

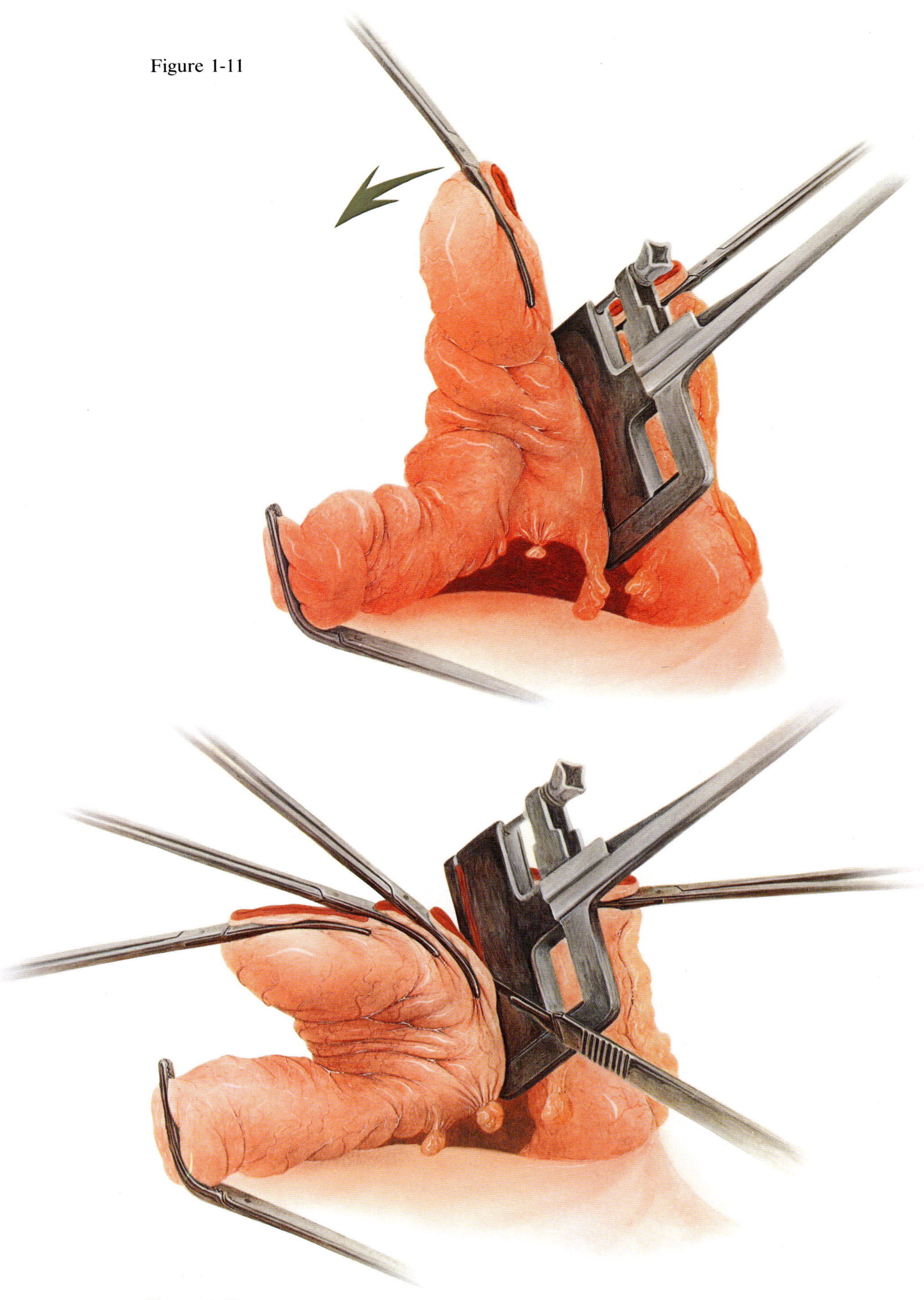

Figure 1-12

Figure 1-13

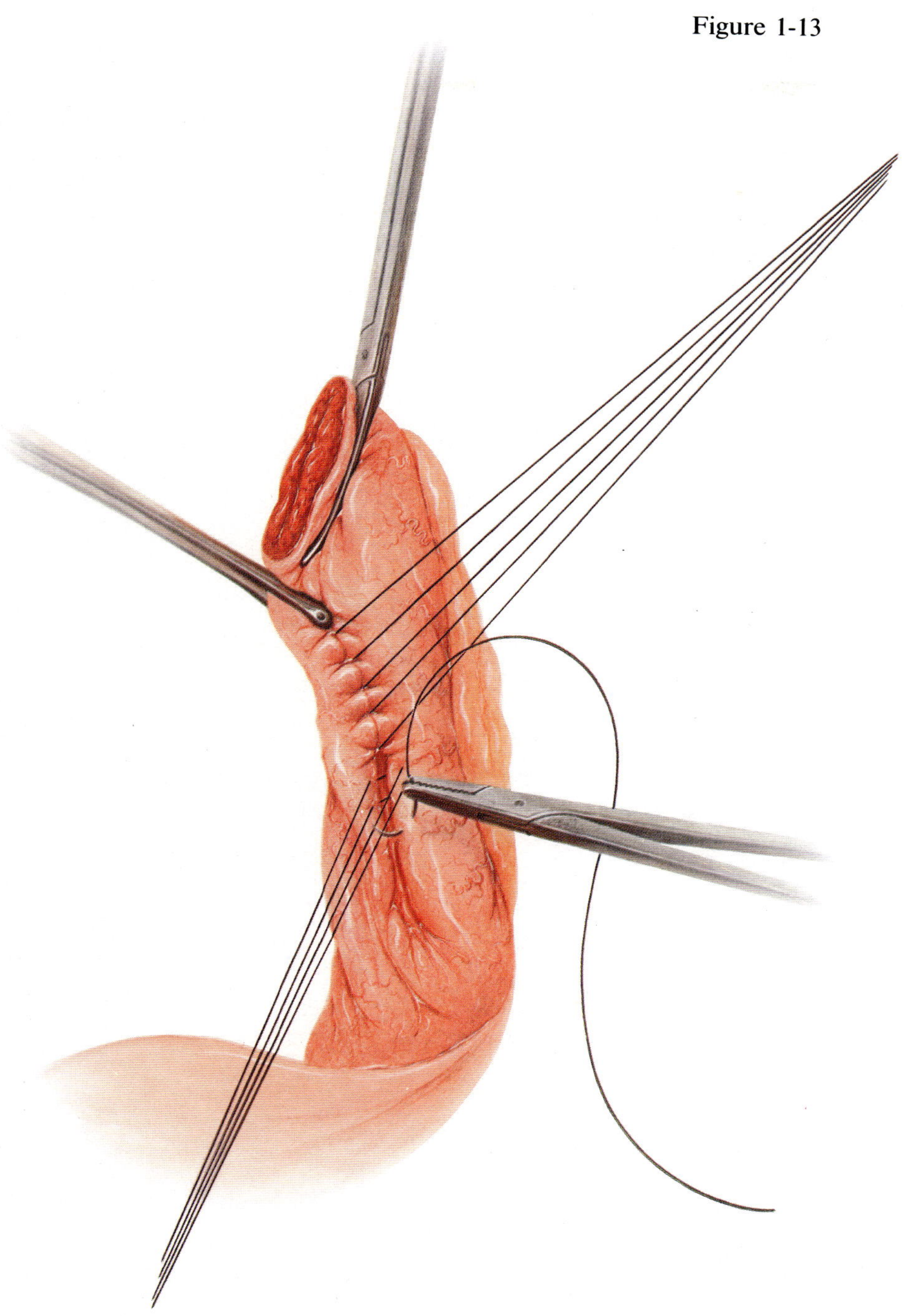

row of interrupted seromuscular silk sutures (Fig. 1-13). When this step is completed (Fig. 1-14), the tubed stomach is grasped with a noncrushing, soft-fabric-shod Foss clamp, and the crushed tissue held in the curved clamps is excised. Again, note the tailoring suture line on the lesser curvature and the right gastroepiploic vessels coursing along the greater curvature of the stomach.

Anastomosis of the cut end of the stomach and the esophagus is then begun (Fig. 1-15); the Foss clamps are widely separated while the sutures are placed. A magnetic mat holds the suture clamps in place so they do not become disorganized. The back, outer row of silk sutures is placed as a horizontal mattress on the stomach side and as a vertical mattress on the esophageal side to make up for the disparity in the sizes of the stomach and esophagus. After all five of the silk sutures are placed (Fig. 1-16), the Foss clamps are brought into parallel apposition, and the row of silk sutures is tied. A running lock stitch of chromic catgut (not shown) effects circumferential mucosal closure. At this point, the Foss clamps are removed, and a 50-F Maloney dilator is passed from the mouth through the anastomotic site. With this dilator in place, the anterior row of interrupted seromuscular sutures is placed and tied (Fig. 1-17). The Maloney dilator acts as a mandrel to ensure adequate caliber of the anastomosis as it is completed.

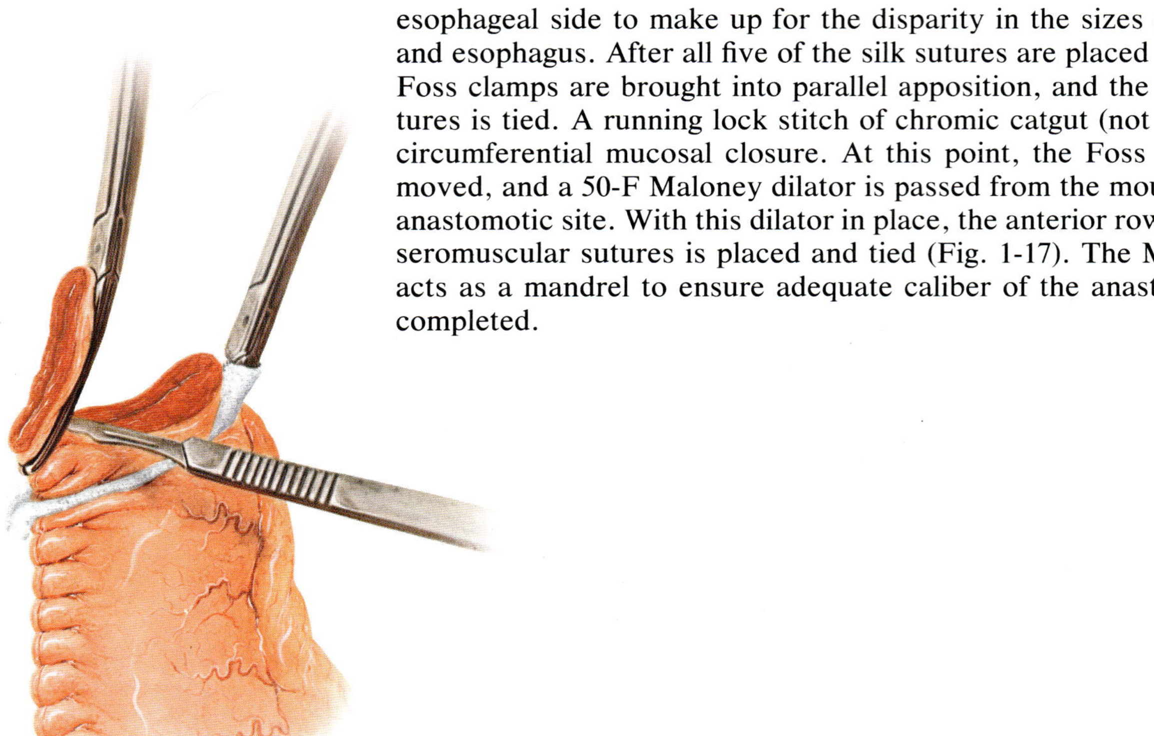

Figure 1-14

Figure 1-15

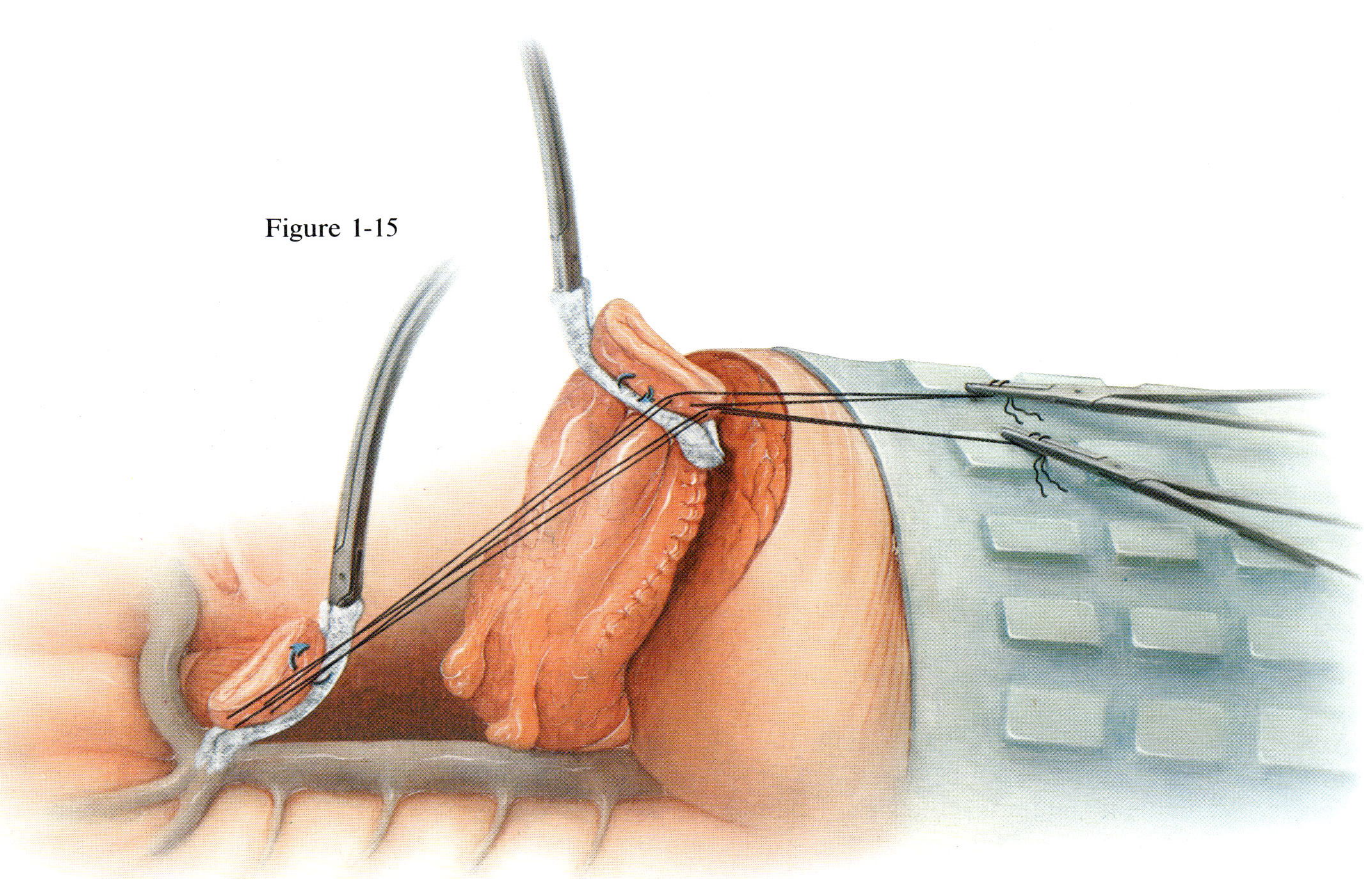

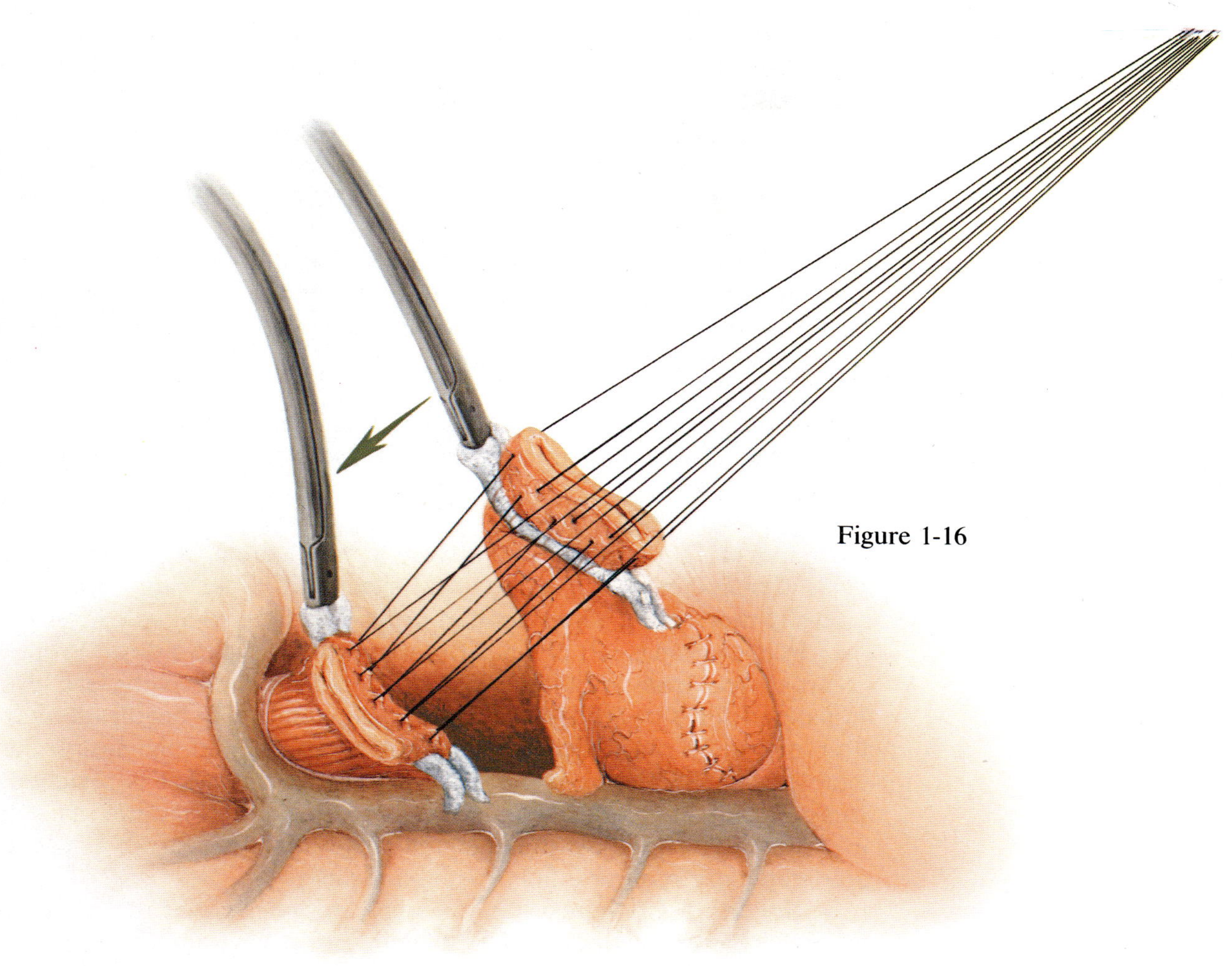

Figure 1-16

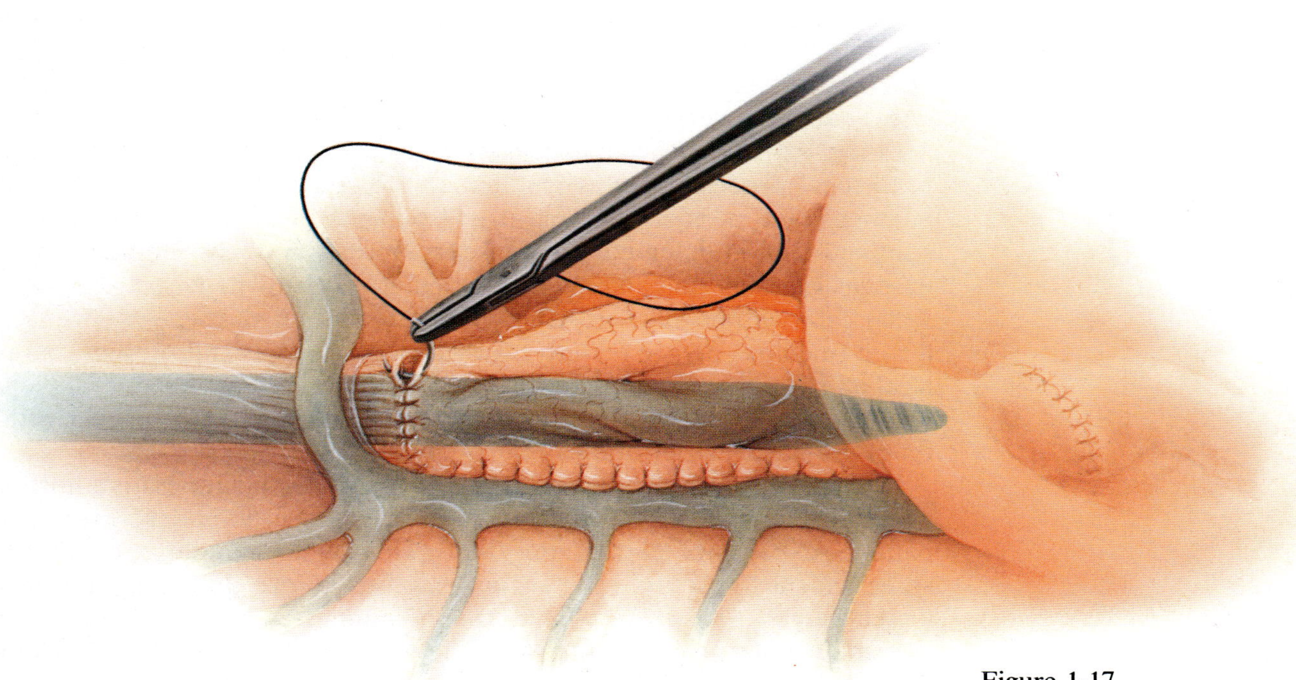

Figure 1-17

The stomach is sutured to the mediastinal pleura along the lesser curvature to relieve any anastomotic tension. The Maloney dilator is removed, and a nasogastric tube is positioned in the stomach.

The chest incision is closed in layers with absorbable suture material. A single 28-F chest catheter is brought from the right pleural space to the outside through a separate stab wound for postoperative suction drainage. A light dressing is applied.

The patient is then turned to the supine position. Because the left pleural space is almost always entered during the course of the procedure and a certain amount of fluid will have accumulated on the left, a single intercostal chest tube is inserted in the fifth or sixth left intercostal space for drainage.

With the patient in a slight Trendelenburg position, a right subclavian venous line is advanced into the superior vena cava for parenteral alimentation.

Postoperative Care. Postoperatively, patients are best managed in a surgical intensive care unit where vital signs and intake and output can be carefully monitored. The retention urinary catheter that was inserted just prior to operation is left in place for approximately 4 to 5 days. Prophylactic broad-spectrum antibiotics, administered preoperatively, are also administered for 4 or 5 days. Parenteral alimentation is begun the morning after operation and is continued until a general diet by mouth can be established. Cimetidine is given intravenously until diet is resumed. All dressings are removed the day after operation. The bilateral chest tubes are removed as soon as drainage and air leaks have ceased. Chest roentgenograms are required daily for monitoring.

On the fifth or sixth postoperative day, evidence of the return of intestinal activity is usually noted. At that point, a Gastrografin contrast esophageal roentgenogram is obtained to check fluoroscopically for anastomotic leak and patency. Prompt diarrheal bowel action usually follows and is further evidence of gastrointestinal patency and readiness for oral dietary intake. If no evidence of an anastomotic leak is found, an oral diet of clear liquids is instituted, and this diet progresses to a general diet during the ensuing 72 hours. Parenteral alimentation is tapered and discontinued as oral intake is established. When the patient is freed of all tubes and venous lines, daily showering and shampooing are encouraged.

In our experience, esophageal leakage, if present, is invariably a confined local process when it is detected radiographically early during the postoperative period. Feeding at this point is disastrous. Thus, when a confined leak is detected, suction decompression of the stomach with a nasogastric tube and parenteral alimentation, with delivery of 2,000 to 3,000 calories per day, are continued. An additional 2 weeks is then allowed to elapse before restudy. If evidence of leak is still present, parenteral alimentation is continued for a total of 3 weeks before an oral diet is resumed. If nasogastric drainage stops or becomes minimal during this time, the nasogastric tube can be safely removed.

Under normal circumstances, an uncomplicated postoperative hospital course is completed in 10 to 14 days. With the operation described, most patients experience early satiety with eating and invariably experience some weight loss during the ensuing months before stabilizing at a new, lesser weight. These effects can often be minimized by having the patient eat small frequent meals during the day and by restricting fluid intake to the periods between meals. With the entire stomach brought into the chest and the esophageal anastomosis at the level of the azygos vein or above, gastroesophageal reflux has not been a problem postoperatively even though an antireflux procedure is not included at the time of operation. Most patients are able to resume full and normal activities approximately 6 weeks from the date of operation.

Total Gastrectomy (Roux-Y)

Technique. The procedure is carried out with the patient under general anesthesia, in the right posterior oblique decubitus position, and stabilized in position with bolsters. The entire left side of the chest and abdomen are prepared and draped into the surgical field. A left thoracoabdominal incision is made, and the pleural space is entered through the bed of the left nonresected eighth rib (seventh intercostal space). This incision is extended across the costal arch and the upper abdomen to the midline, and it ends at a point halfway between the naval and xiphoid. The costal arch is divided with a bone shears, and the cartilaginous arch is trimmed flush with the seventh and eighth ribs. The diaphragm is incised radially 8 to 10 cm, and the diaphragmatic vessels are sutured and ligated as they are divided. This diaphragmatic incision permits the rib incision to be spread with a self-retaining retractor to expose the distal esophagus and viscera of the left upper quadrant.

In practice, one actually explores the abdomen through the abdominal limb of the thoracoabdominal incision to determine resectability before the described incision is completed. If resection is not possible, a palliative Celestin tube, if applicable, can be inserted.

With the exposure provided by the described thoracoabdominal incision, one can effect total gastrectomy with distal esophagectomy and reconstruction without further positioning or incision. The steps of the resective phase of the procedure, which has the same anatomic format as other procedures, are shown in Figure 1-18.

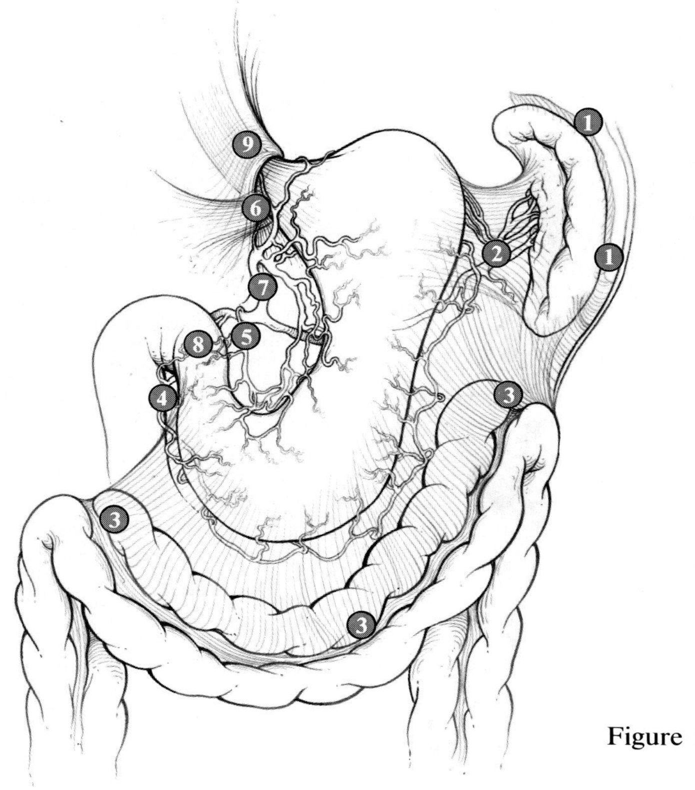

Figure 1-18

Figure 1-19

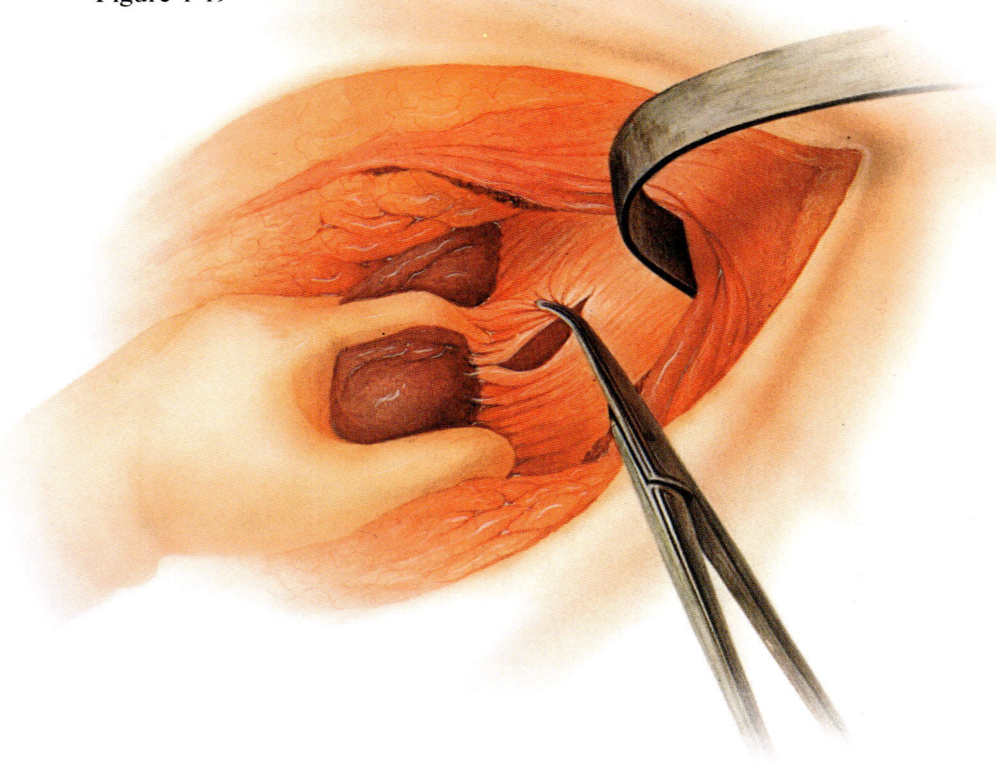

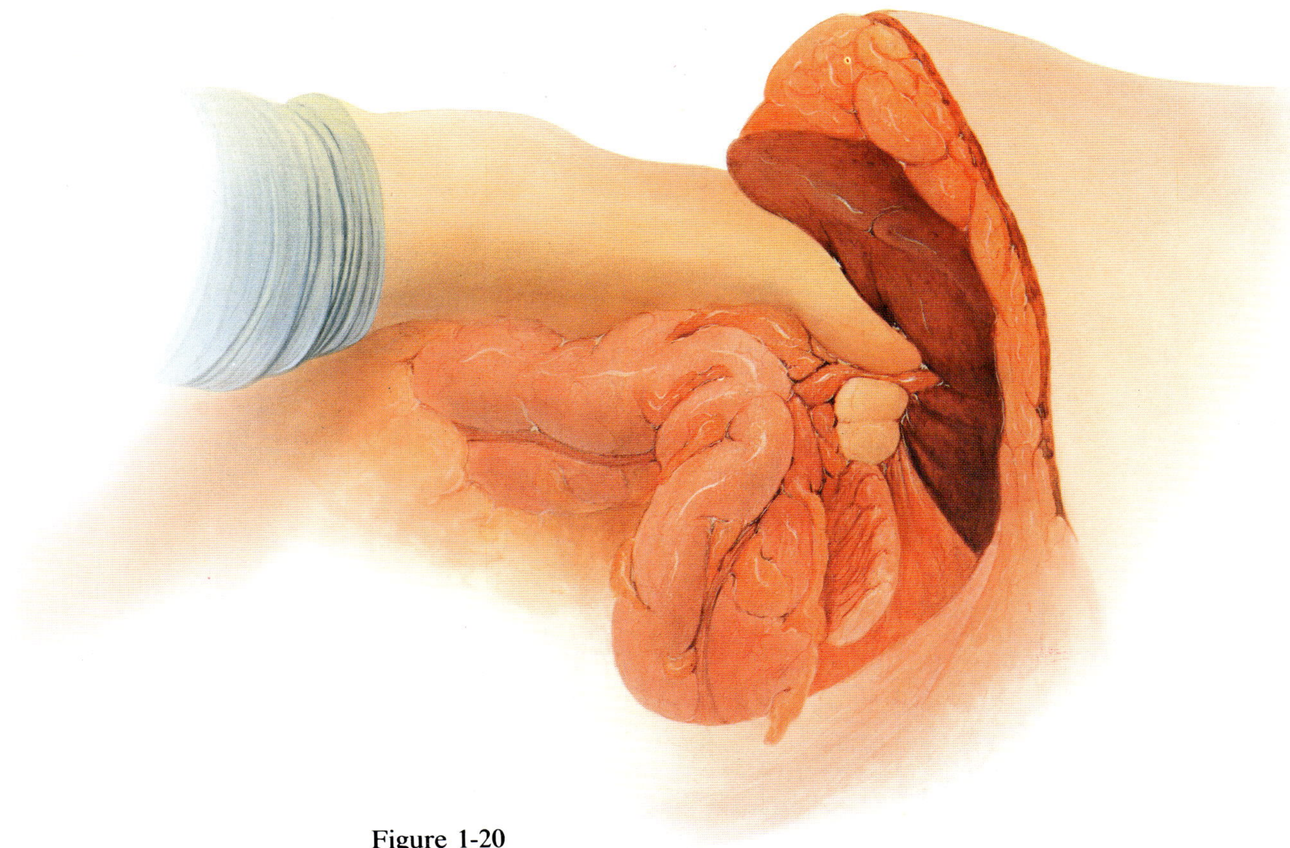

Figure 1-20

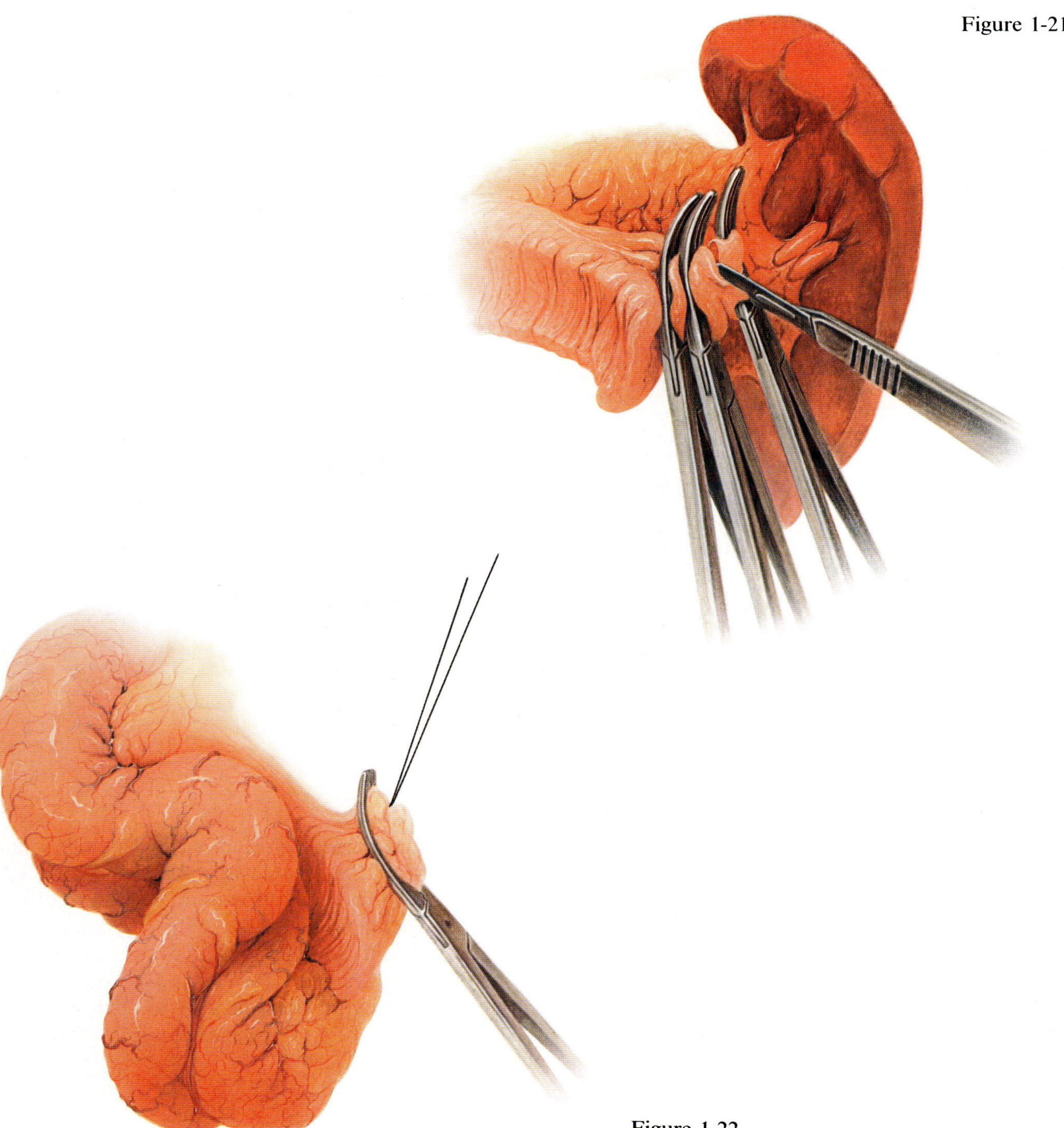

Figure 1-21

Figure 1-22

With the exposure afforded by the left thoracoabdominal incision, Step 1, mobilization of the spleen, is effected by incising the peritoneum lateral to the splenic hilus beneath the diaphragm. This lienorenal incision (Fig. 1-19) permits the spleen and tail of the pancreas to be lifted ventrally off the perirenal fat. Step 2, interruption of the splenic vessels, leaves the spleen attached to the stomach by short gastric vessels. This step is accomplished initially by blunt dissection to encircle the splenic vessels at the splenic hilus with the hand (Fig. 1-20). This maneuver then permits the application of clamps to the splenic hilar vessels for division (Fig. 1-21) and subsequent double ligation of the splenic vessels (Fig. 1-22).

Figure 1-23

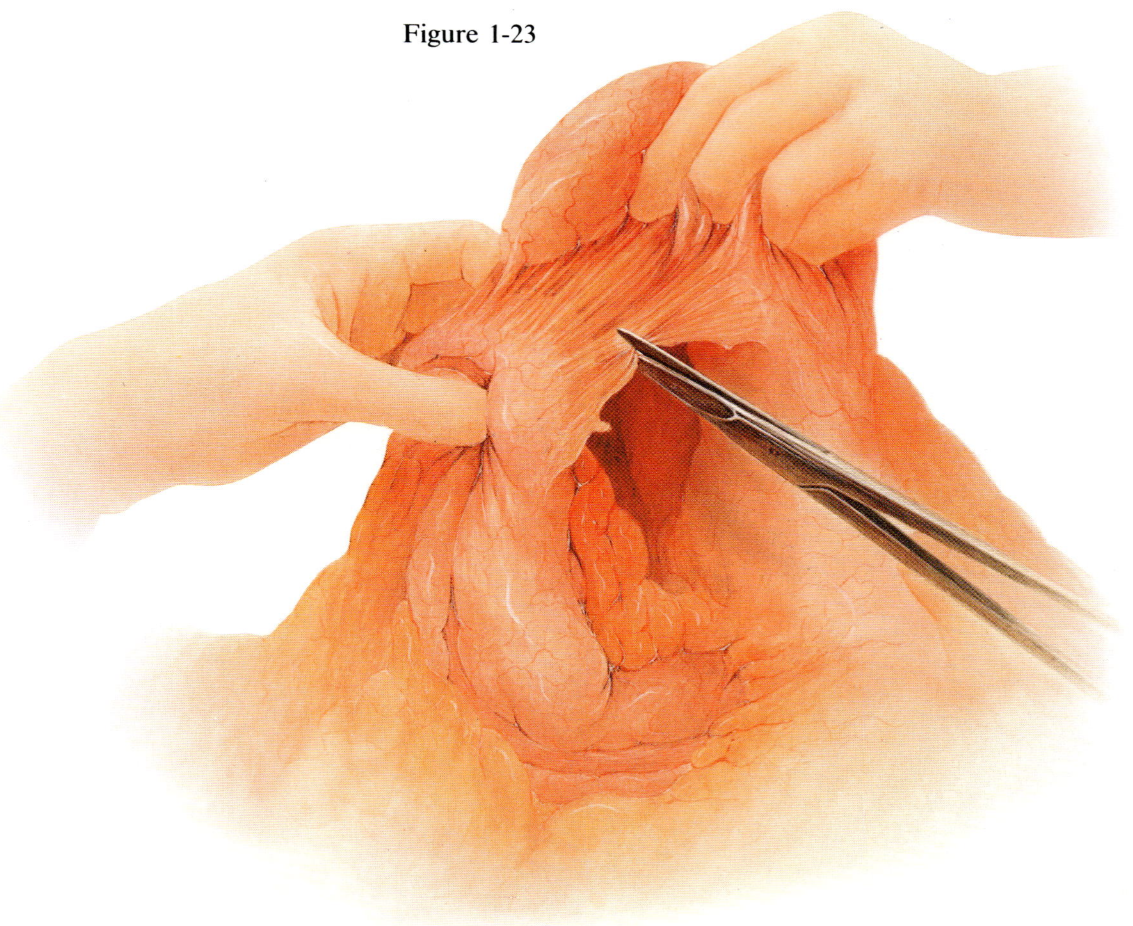

Step 3, disconnection of the greater omentum from the transverse colon, extends from the hepatic flexure to the splenic flexure (Fig. 1-23). The anatomic details that make separation of the omentum from the colon a relatively simple maneuver are shown in Fig. 1-24. With cephalad reflection of the pendulous omental apron, the thin avascular connections between the omentum and colon are visualized for sharp division. Steps 4 and 5 entail the interruption and ligation of the distal blood supply to the stomach, specifically the right gastric and right gastroepiploic vessels.

Figure 1-24

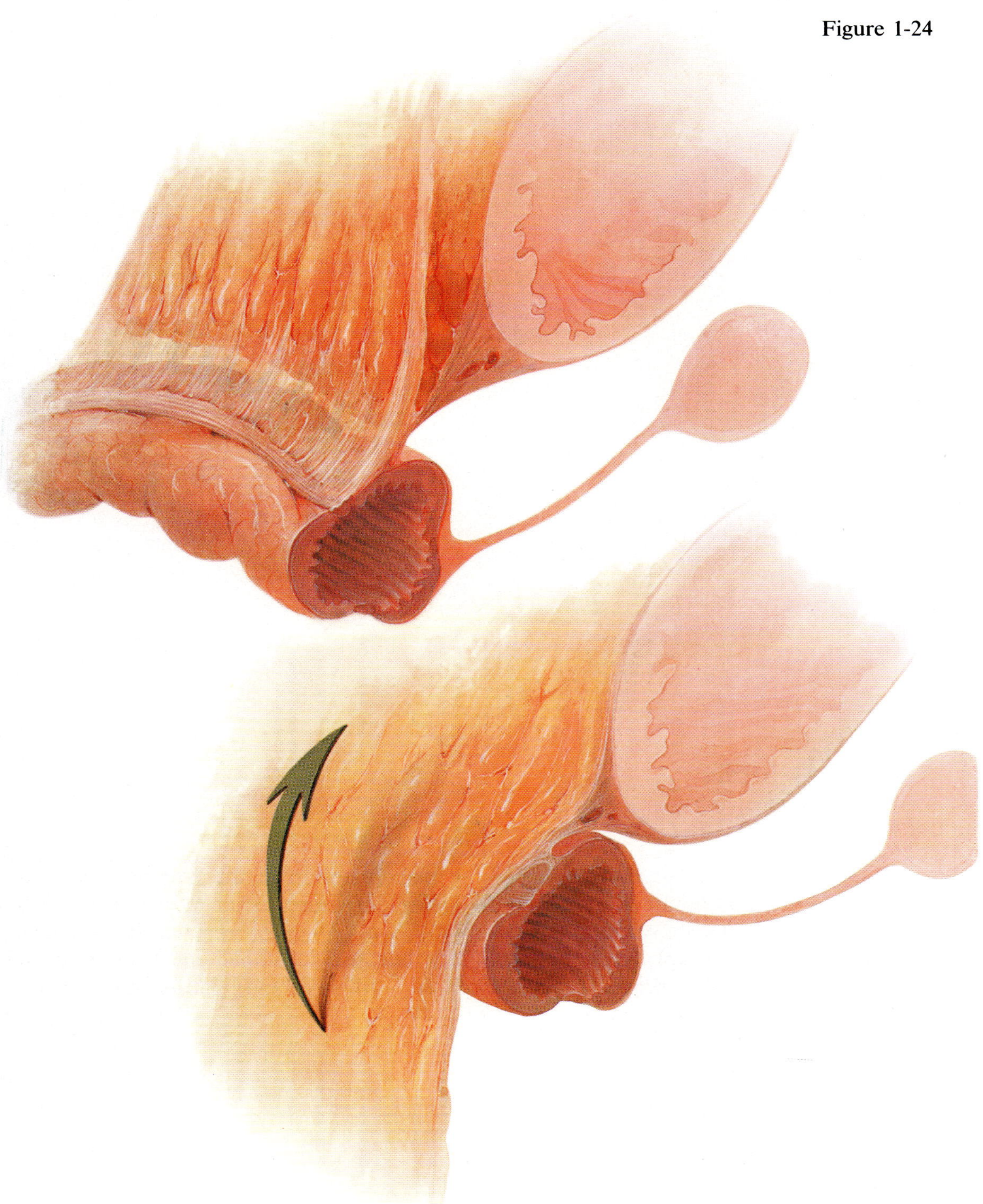

Figure 1-25

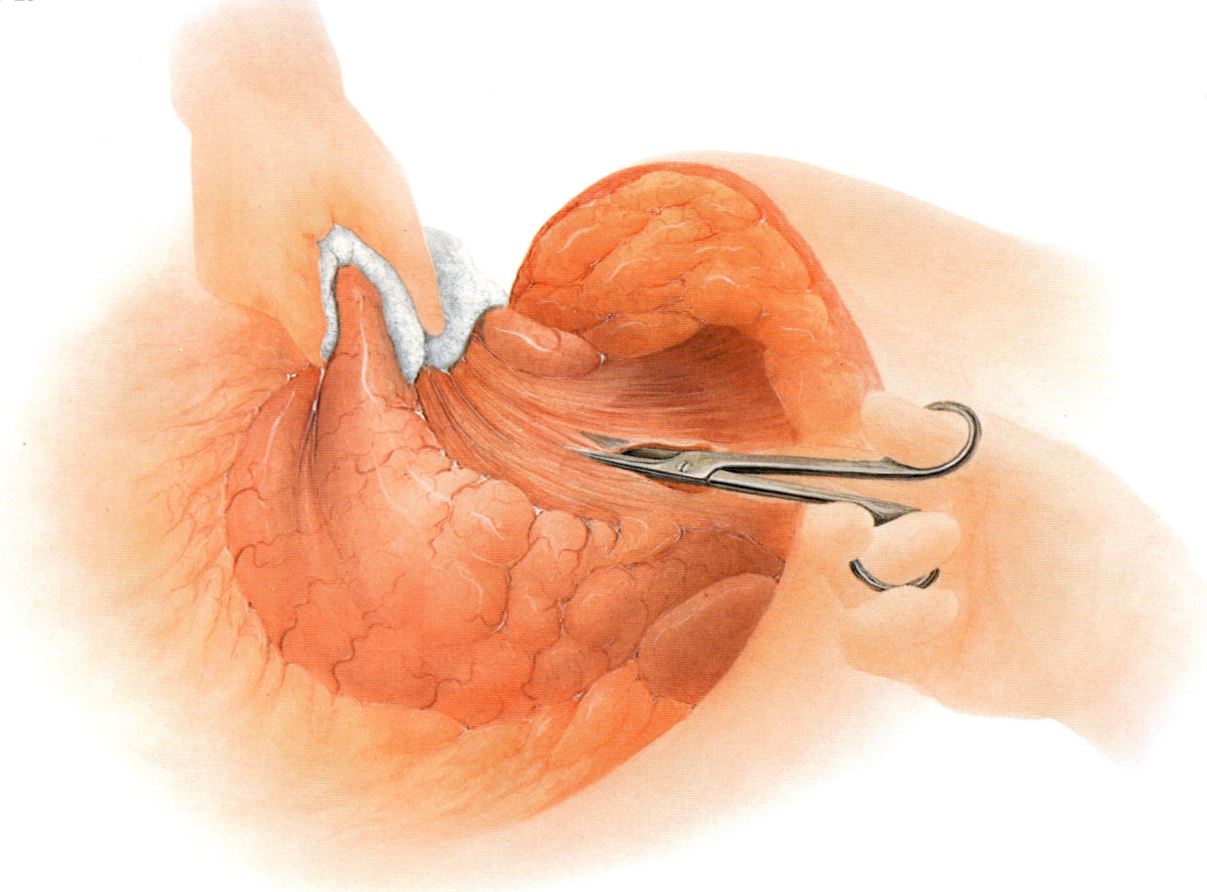

Step 6 is continuation of the disconnection of the stomach from the parietal connections along the lesser curvature. After interruption of the right gastric vessels, the lower, rather attenuated, avascular lesser omentum is simply incised (Fig. 1-25); because its upper end is thicker and vascular, it requires formal clamping, division, and ligation of the gastrohepatic omentum (Fig. 1-26).

Figure 1-26

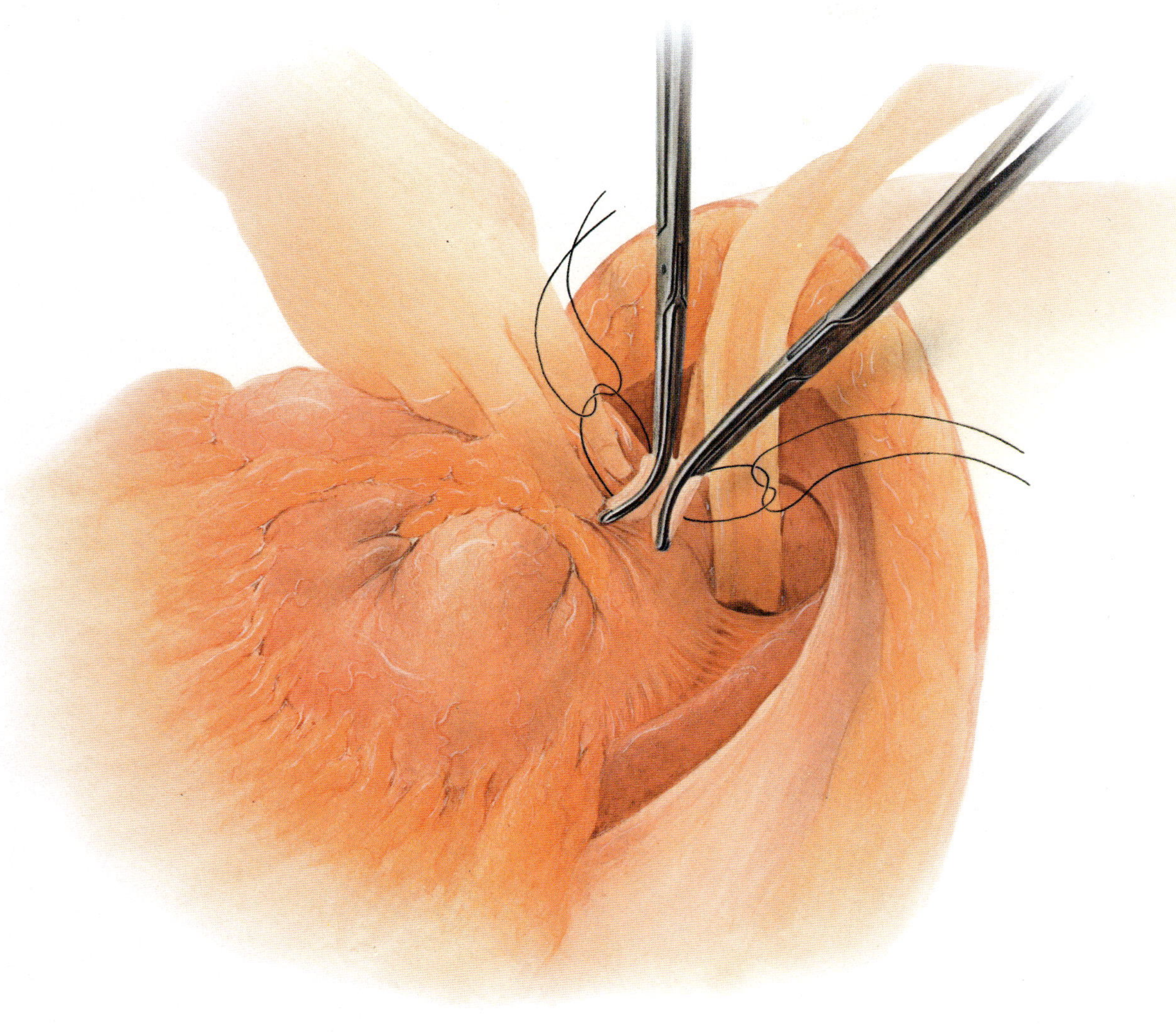

Figure 1-27

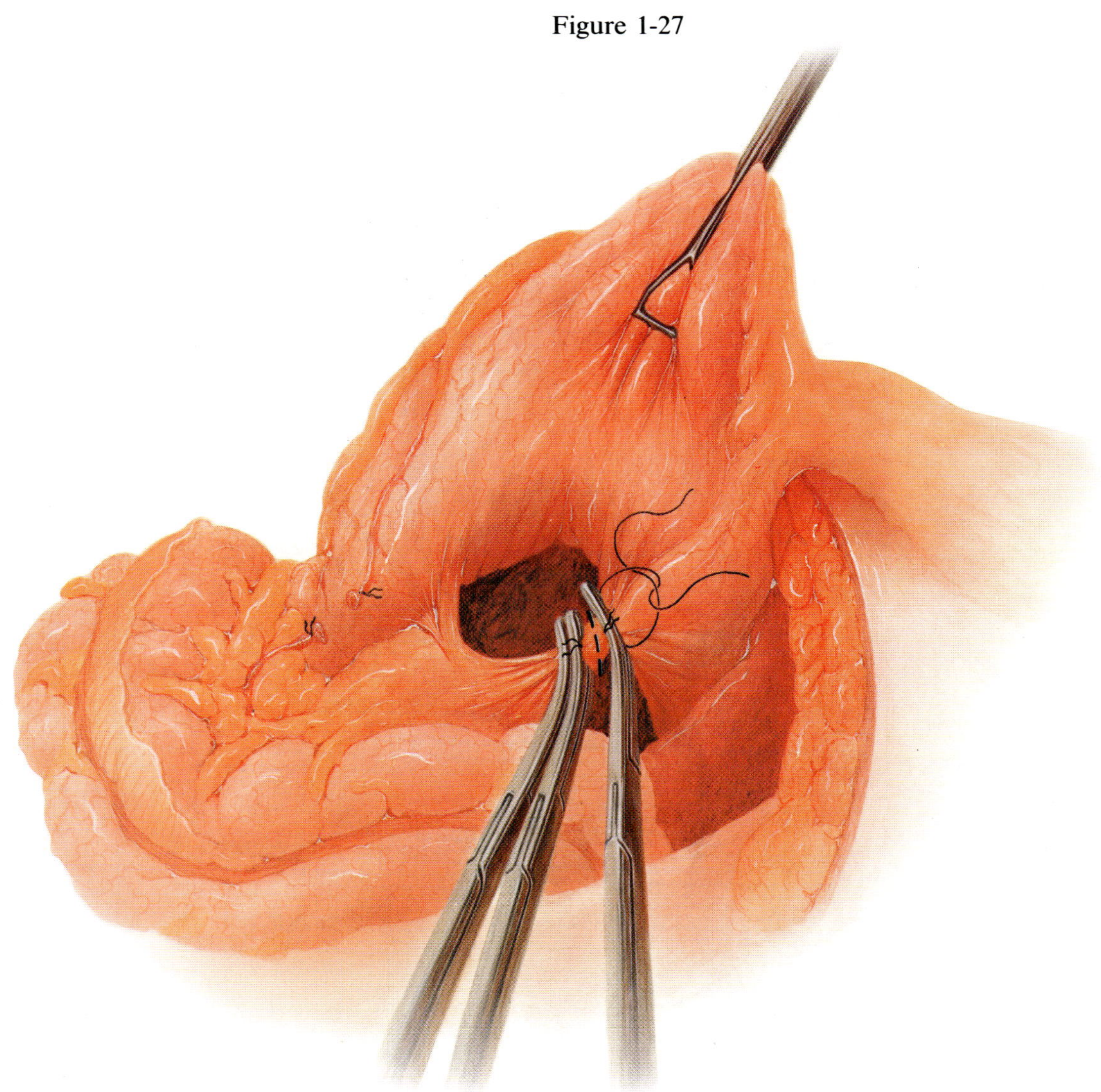

Step 7 is interruption of the left gastric vessels, the final vascular connection to the stomach. This step is best effected with cephalad reflection of the greater curvature of the stomach and isolation of the vessels behind the stomach through the lesser sac (Fig. 1-27). Step 8 is transection and closure of the duodenum with a TA 30 stapling device just distal to a curved clamp placed just beyond the pylorus (Fig. 1-28). The row of staples on the duodenal stump is buried beneath a row of interrupted seromuscular sutures.

Figure 1-28

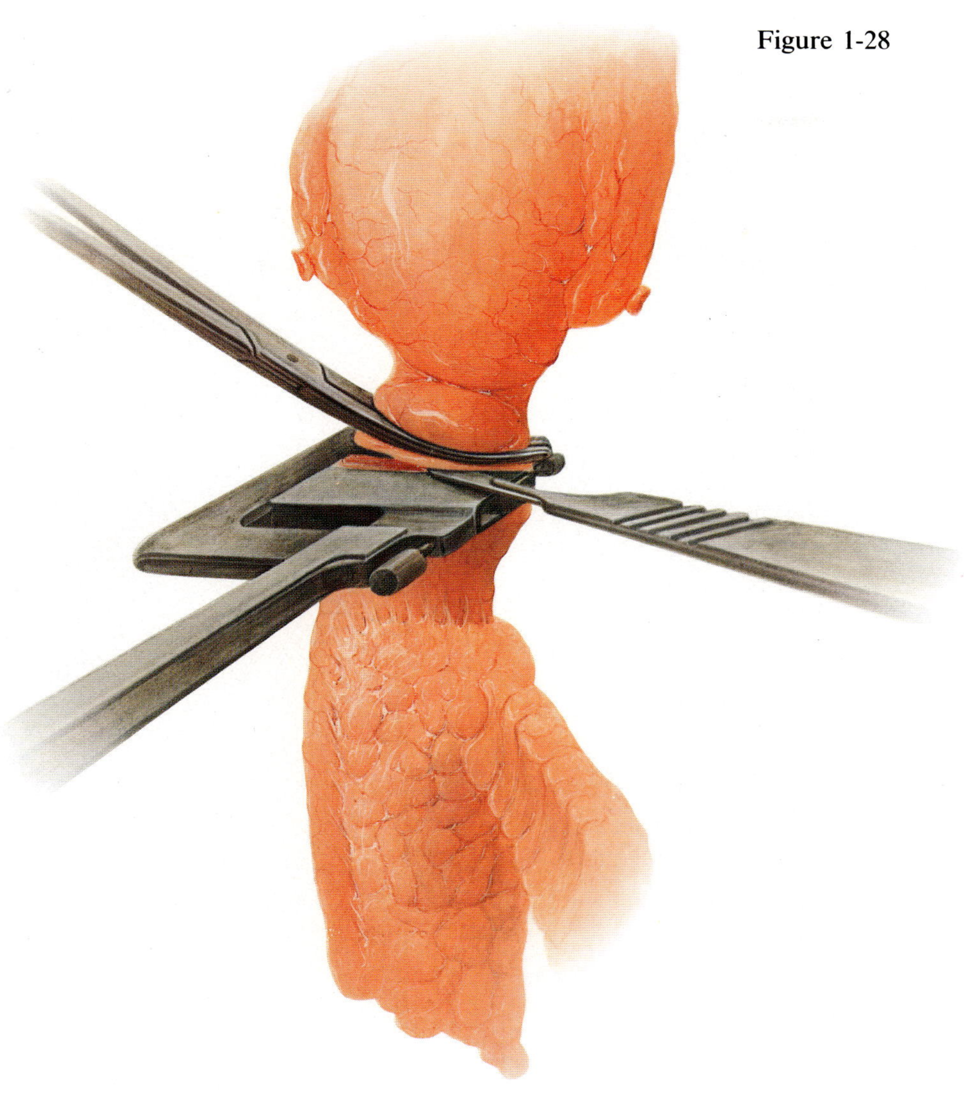

Figure 1-29

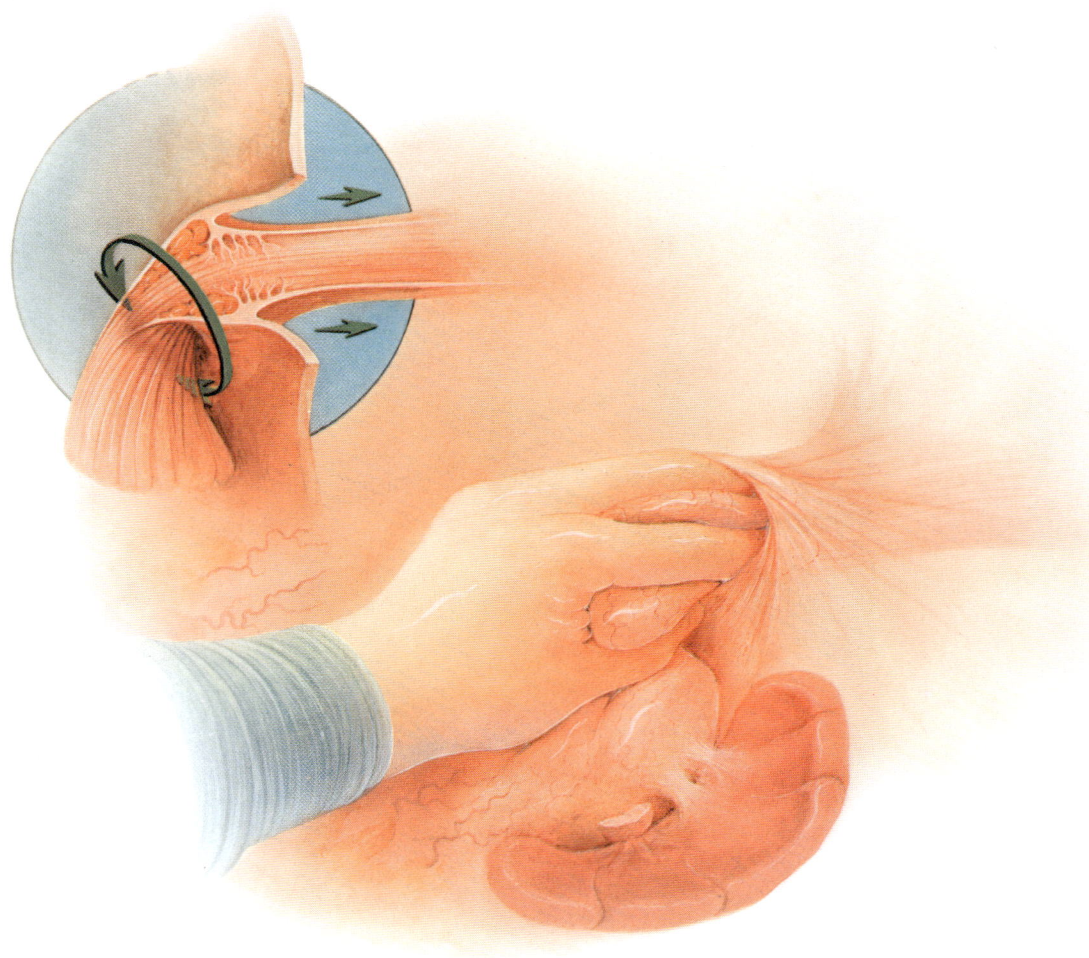

Step 9 is the final maneuver of the resective phase. It entails mobilization of the distal esophagus for transection well above the tumor. In the chest, it involves division of the left inferior pulmonary ligament, which permits the lung to be retracted cephalad. A Penrose drain is passed around the lower esophagus and vagi to elevate them from the posterior mediastinum (see Fig. 1-44). On the abdominal side of the esophageal hiatus, the distal esophagus is encircled and bluntly dissected free of all diaphragmatic attachments (Fig. 1-29). On rare occasions, neoplastic fixation to the crus will require actual excision of a cuff of diaphragm that is left attached to the esophagus. A Foss clamp is applied to the esophagus 8 to 10 cm above the esophagogastric junction in the chest (Fig. 1-30), and the esophagus is transected and closed distally with a TA 30 stapling device.

The final en bloc surgical specimen consists of the distal esophagus, the entire stomach with attached spleen, the greater and lesser omenta, and the rim of duodenum with attached lymph-bearing tissues (Fig. 1-31).

Figure 1-30

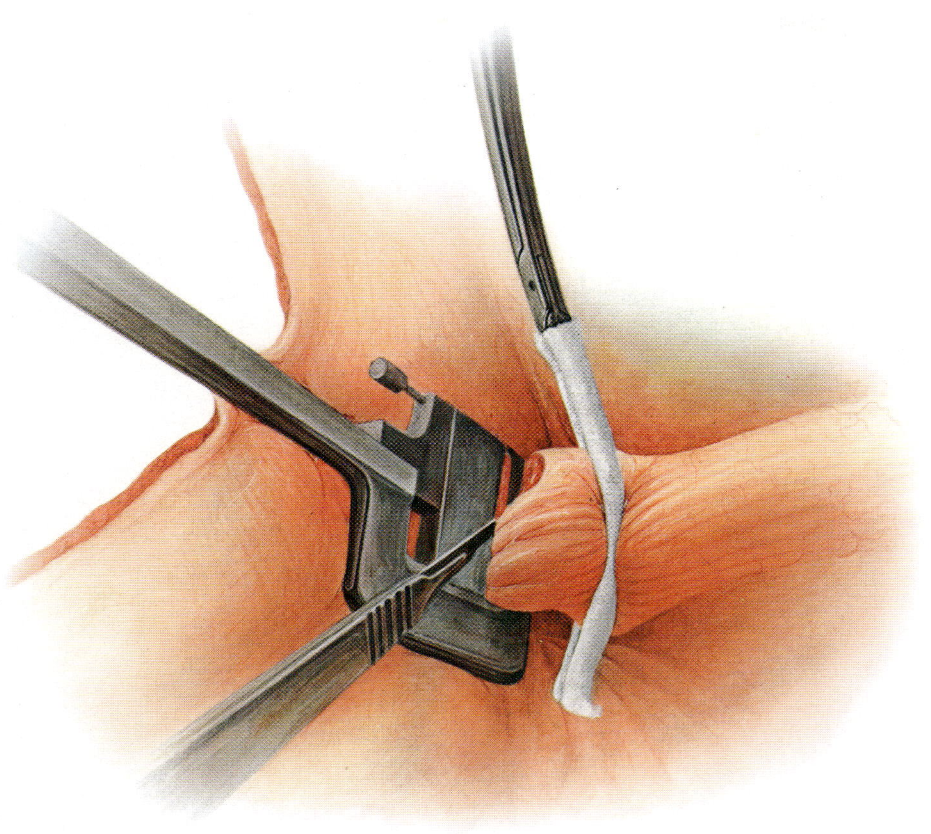

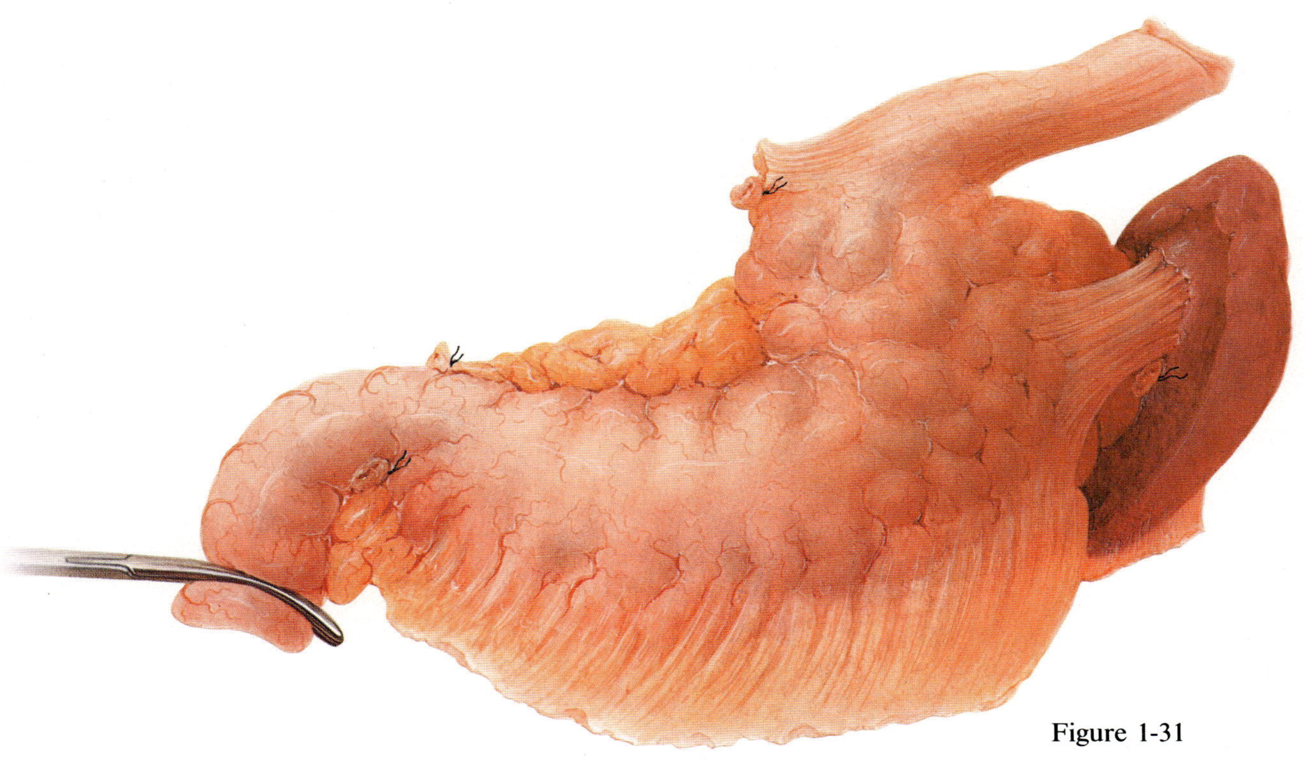

Figure 1-31

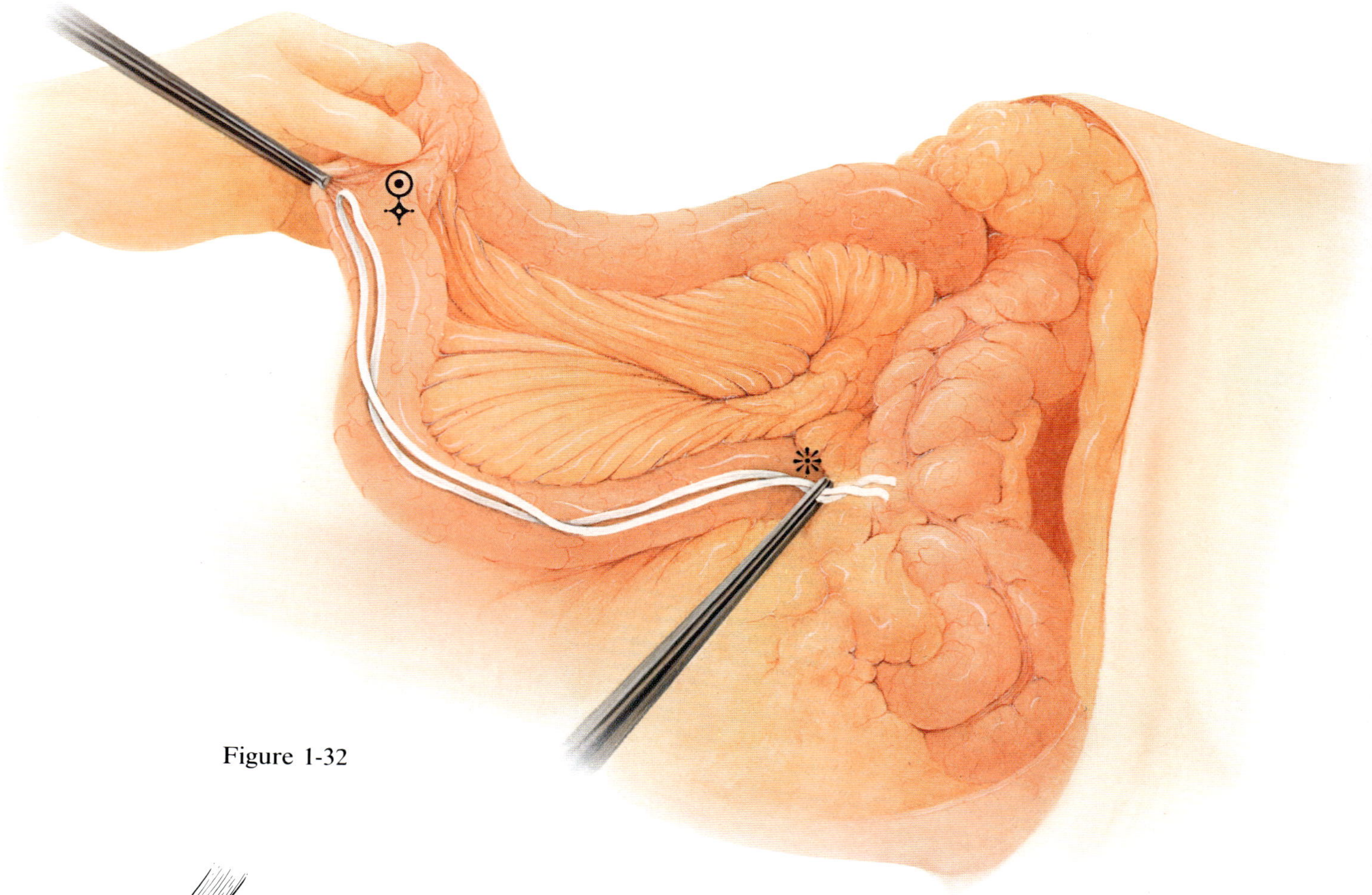

Figure 1-32

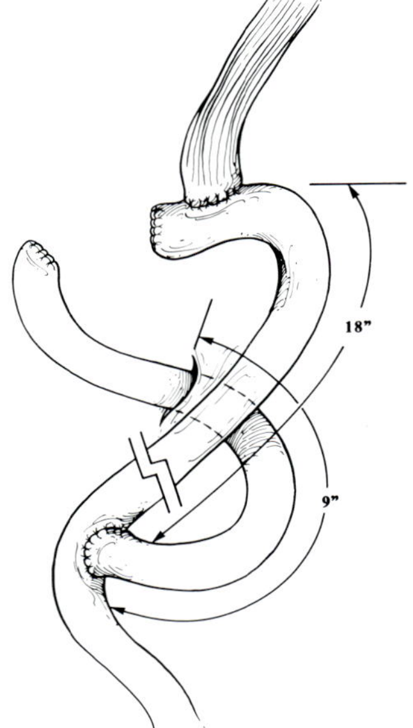

Total Gastrectomy
Roux-Y
Reconstruction

The reconstructive phase is then begun. In essence, it entails the construction of an 18-inch (46-cm) long-limb Roux-Y of jejunum that is anastomosed to the esophagus to restore esophagoenteric continuity.

In the abdomen, the ligament of Treitz is identified. With use of a previously measured tape, a point 9 inches (23 cm) distal to this duodenojejunal junction is determined and marked by placing an Allis forceps on the antimesenteric border of the jejunum (Fig. 1-32). The mesentery of the small bowel is transilluminated to permit precise interruption of the mesenteric vessels as the mesentery is incised radially (Fig. 1-33). The distal jejunal mesentery must also be divided at right angles to the radial incision to develop it as a pedicle with sufficient length to reach the esophagus in the chest.

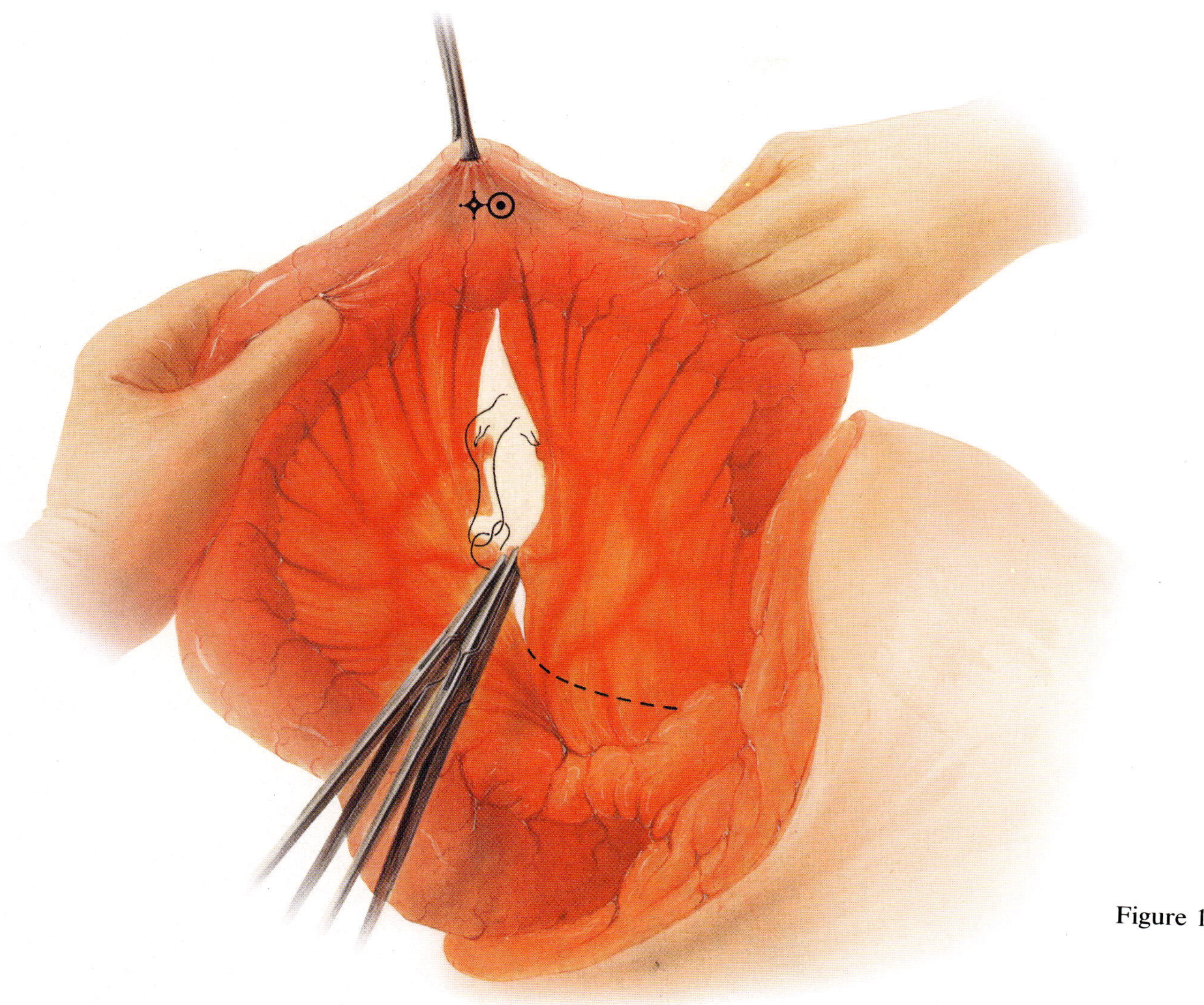

Figure 1-33

Figure 1-34

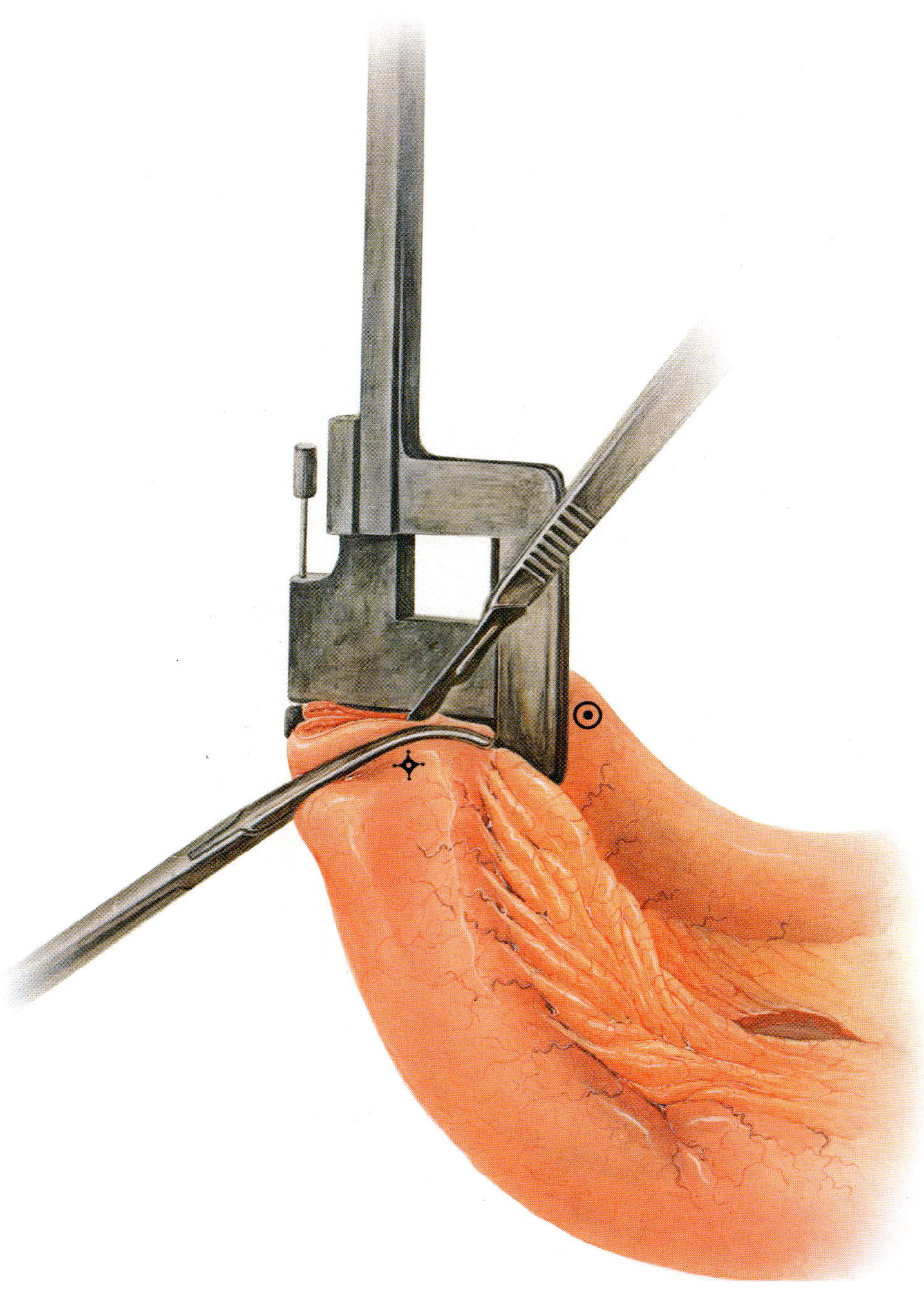

After the jejunal mesentery is divided, the jejunum is divided by using a TA 30 stapling device to close the distal end. A curved clamp is left on the proximal end (Fig. 1-34), and the row of staples is buried beneath a row of interrupted silk sutures (Fig. 1-35).

A defect is made in the transverse mesocolon in an avascular area near the ligament of Treitz (Fig. 1-36). This defect permits the passage of the closed end of the distal jejunum cephalad through the transverse mesocolon and esophageal hiatus to the divided end of the esophagus in the chest.

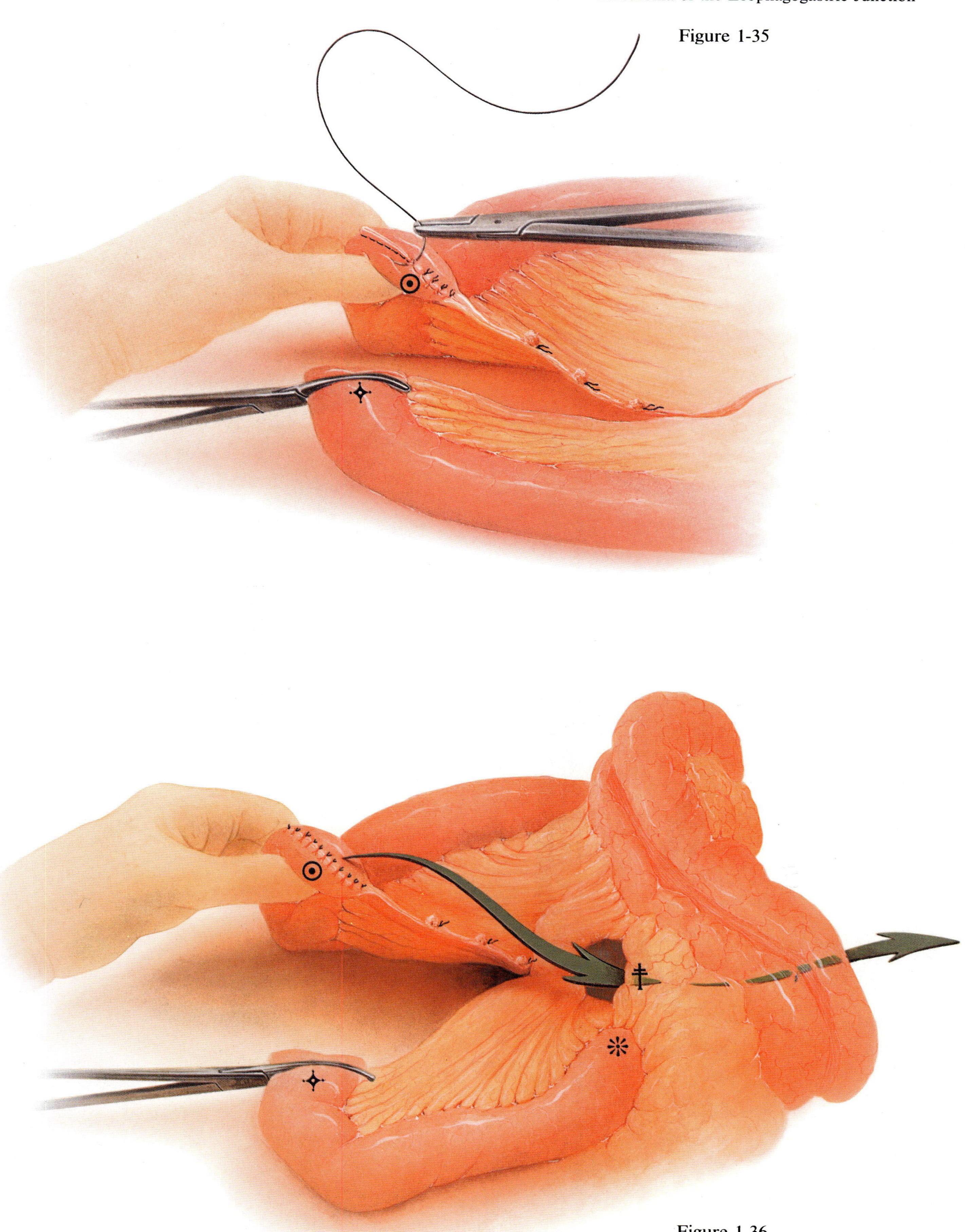

Figure 1-35

Figure 1-36

Figure 1-37

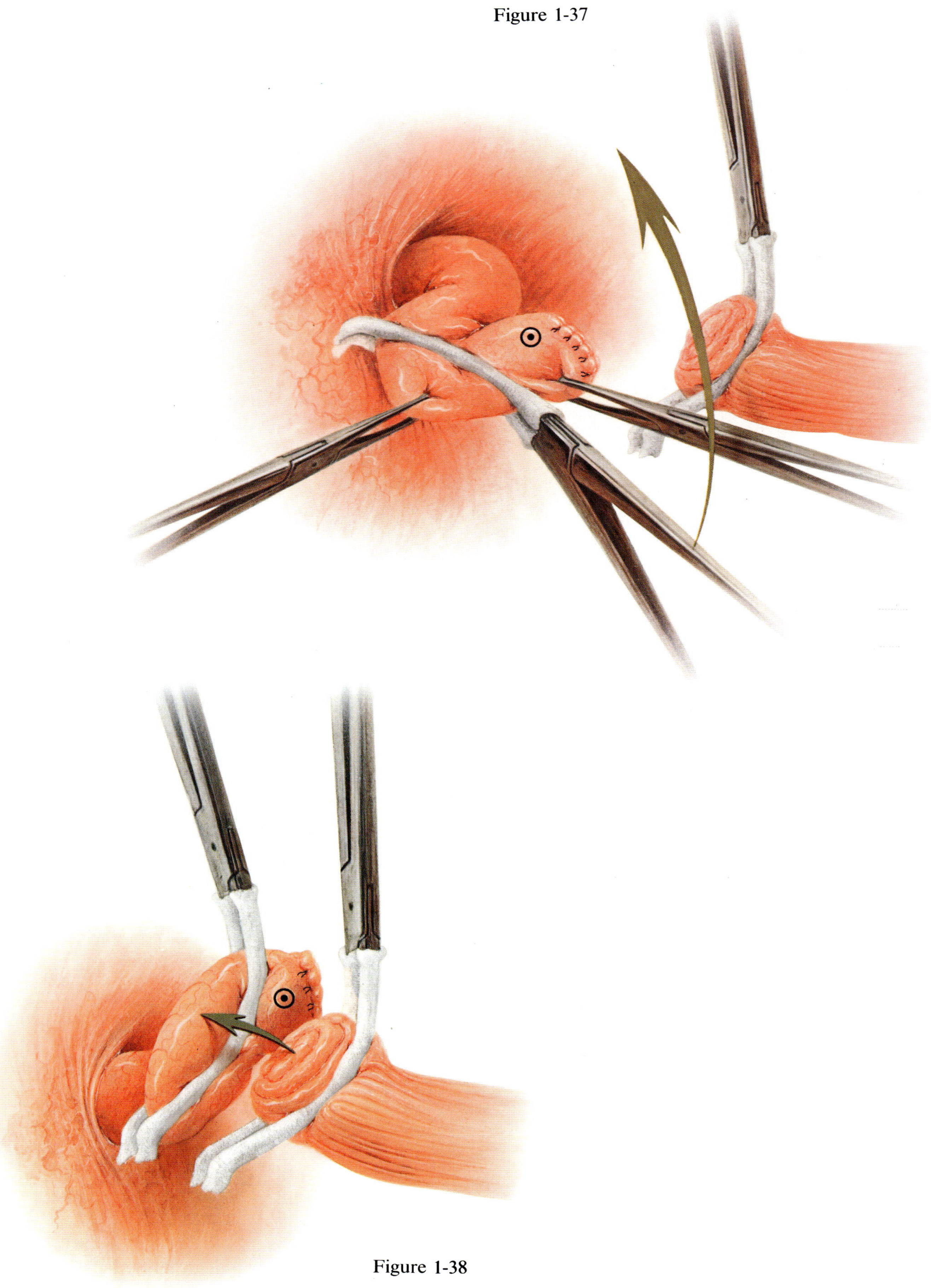

Figure 1-38

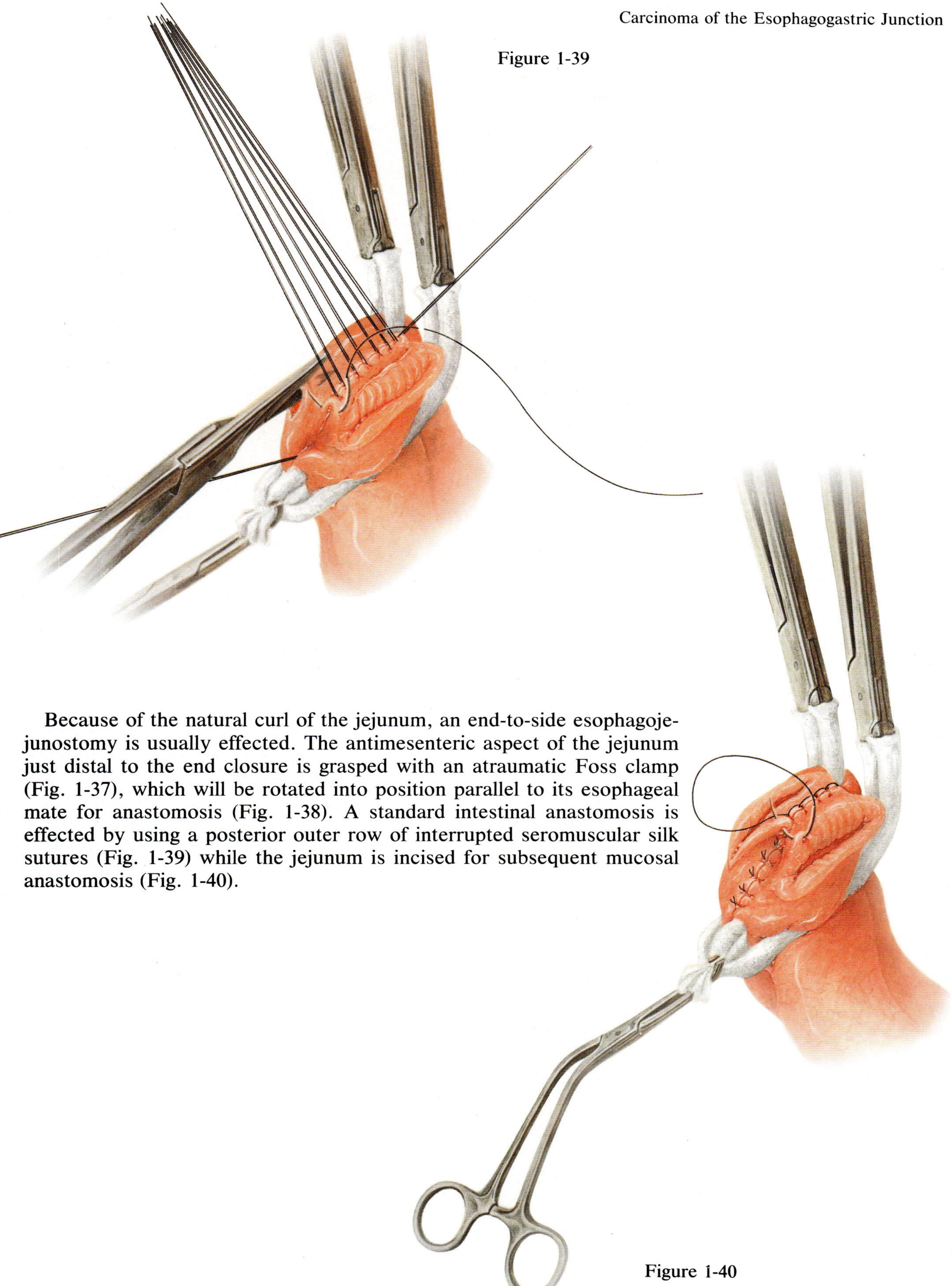

Figure 1-39

Because of the natural curl of the jejunum, an end-to-side esophagojejunostomy is usually effected. The antimesenteric aspect of the jejunum just distal to the end closure is grasped with an atraumatic Foss clamp (Fig. 1-37), which will be rotated into position parallel to its esophageal mate for anastomosis (Fig. 1-38). A standard intestinal anastomosis is effected by using a posterior outer row of interrupted seromuscular silk sutures (Fig. 1-39) while the jejunum is incised for subsequent mucosal anastomosis (Fig. 1-40).

Figure 1-40

Figure 1-41

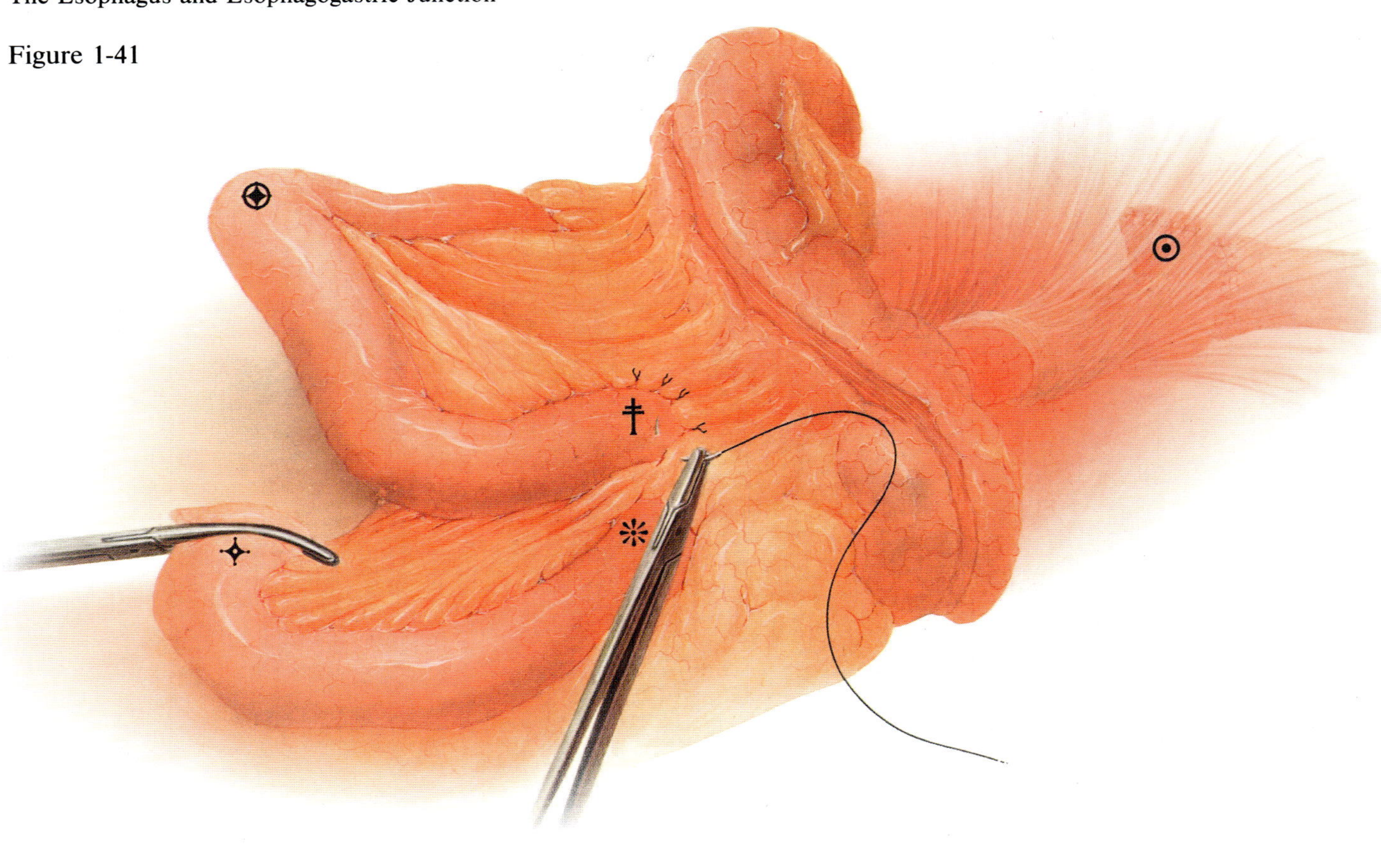

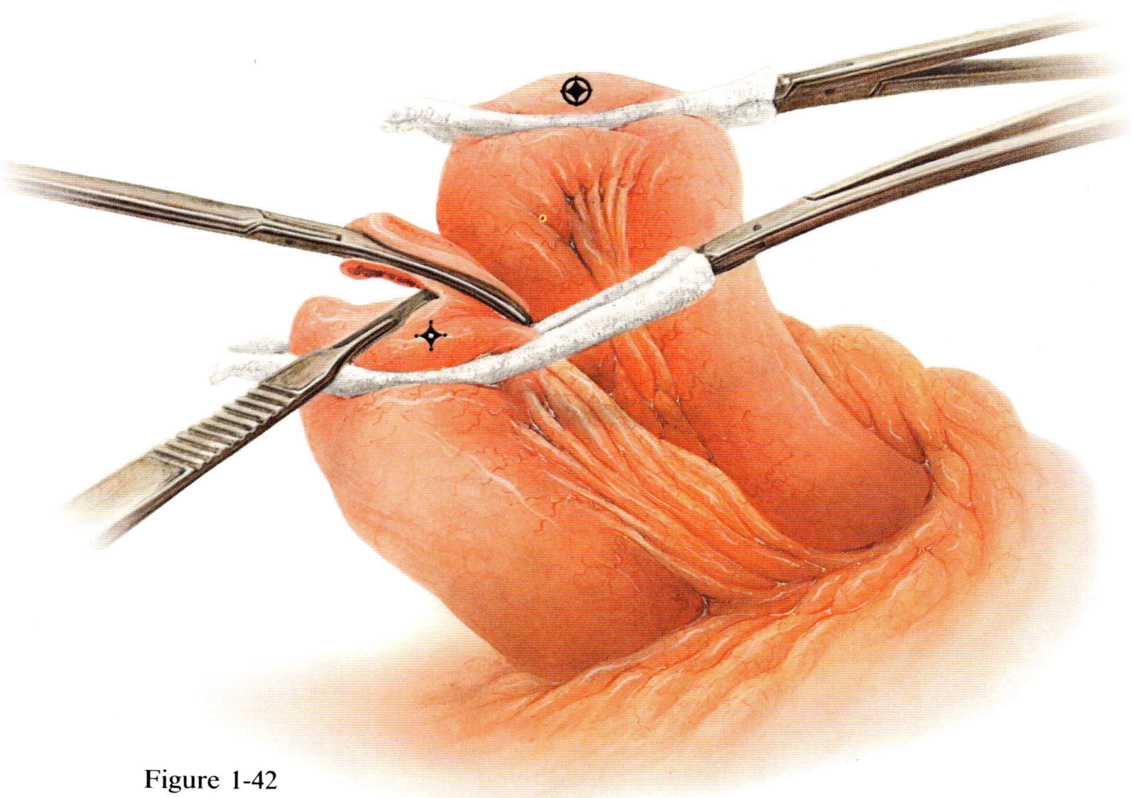

Figure 1-42

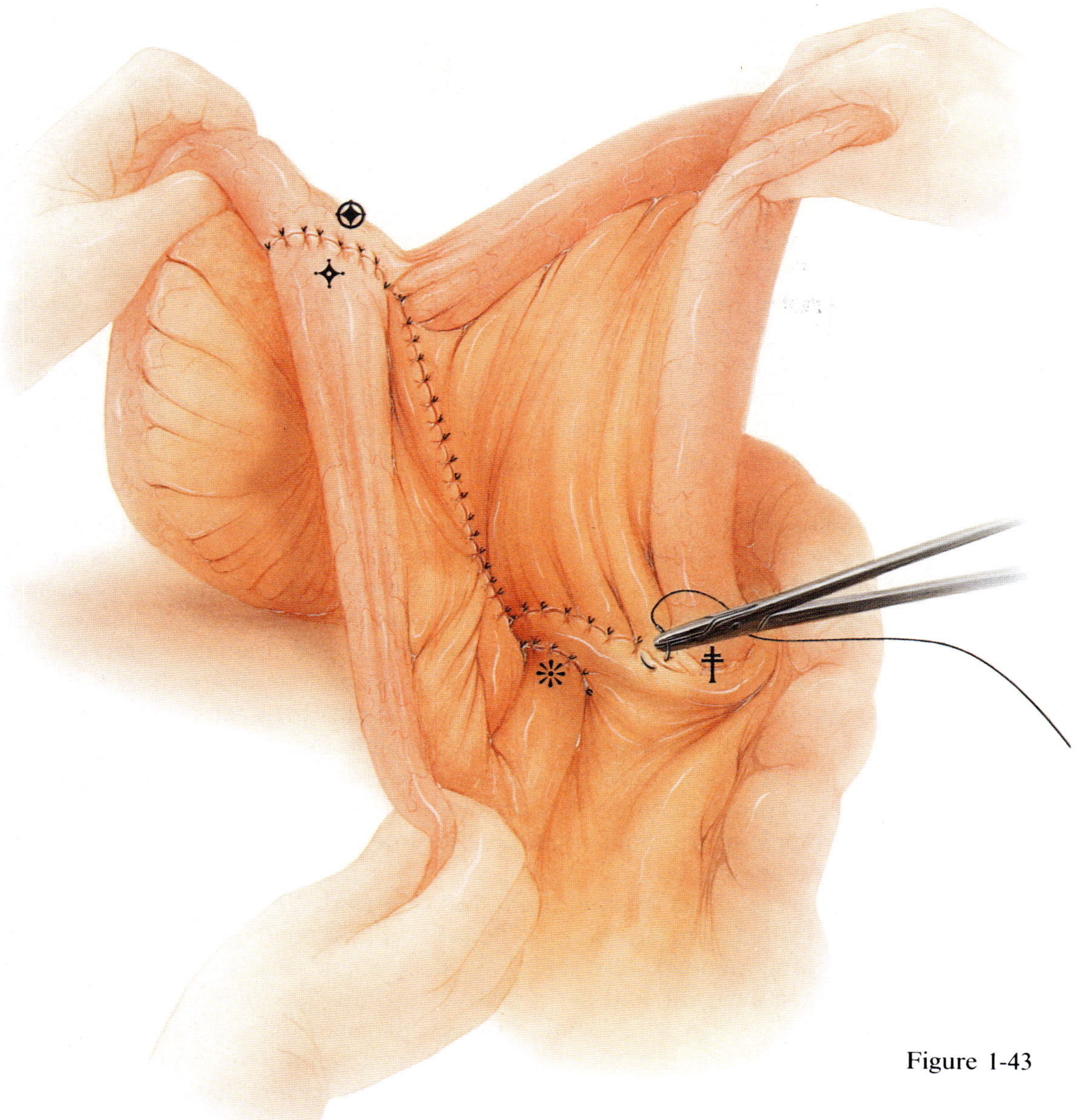

Figure 1-43

The reflux of biliary-pancreatic secretions up the esophagus is prevented by selecting a point 18 inches (46 cm) distal to the esophagojejunostomy for end-to-side jejunojejunostomy (Fig. 1-41). Note that this long limb of jejunum will require suture closure around it at points where it passes through the transverse mesocolon and diaphragm to prevent internal herniation.

End-to-side jejunojejunostomy is effected in a manner identical to esophagojejunostomy (Fig. 1-42) (see also Fig. 1-39 and 1-40).

After completion of the jejunal anastomosis, it is apparent that the intersection of the mesenteric planes leaves defects that are potential sites for internal herniation, and these require suture closure (Fig. 1-43).

A Levin tube is passed through a nostril down the esophagus and through the esophagojejunostomy into the upper part of the jejunum. Two Penrose drains are brought from the abdomen to the outside through an epigastric stab wound; one of the drains leads from the duodenal stump, and the other leads from the esophagojejunostomy through the esophageal hiatus to the outside. A sterile adhesive bag is applied to the drain site to collect drainage and provide an airtight seal. The mediastinal pleura is sutured closed over the lower esophagus and upper jejunum in the chest. The short radial incision in the diaphragm is closed with heavy figure-of-eight Dacron sutures. The ribs are approximated with heavy pericostal sutures of absorbable suture material. A single catheter is brought from the left pleural space to the outside through a separate stab wound. Both the abdominal and the chest wounds are closed in layers with buried and absorbable suture material. A subcutaneous catheter is used to prevent wound infection, after the method of McIlrath.

Postoperative Care. Postoperatively, patients who undergo total gastrectomy are cared for essentially the same as was described for patients who undergo the Ivor-Lewis resection. An exception, of course, is absence of the need for cimetidine after total gastrectomy. Penrose drains are left in place until an oral diet is well established and drainage is minimal. The chief advantage of the 18-inch (46-cm) Roux-Y is that it diverts duodenal contents into the distal jejunum and prevents their reflux into the esophagus, and it thereby provides a comfortable functional result. As with the Ivor-Lewis procedure, early satiety is a regular feature of this operation, but this problem diminishes with time. Regular monthly parenteral vitamin B_{12} supplementation is required after total gastrectomy to prevent megaloblastic anemia.

The results after operations for cancer of the gastric cardia are well established. During the past decade, approximately 90% of our patients have experienced satisfactory swallowing and digestive function throughout their survival, and the operative mortality has decreased from approximately 12% to 8%. Death from esophageal leakage has been virtually eliminated by the measures described. Overall, the 5-year survival remains at 20%. The results are slightly more favorable when lymph nodes are not metastatically involved. Thus, the procedures defined provide good palliation for most patients and are not prejudicial to cure for the few who can have their tumors ablated. Further, they provide restoration of comfortable digestion and nutrition. Overall, they are associated with acceptable morbidity and mortality rates.

Gastroesophageal Reflux and Its Complications

The factors responsible for competence at the gastroesophageal junction were defined in "Physiology," this chapter.

Gastroesophageal incompetence is a consequence of various aberrations. The disorder most often occurs as a consequence of anatomic derangement, notably the sliding esophageal hiatal hernia, which may obliterate an effective segment of intra-abdominal esophagus and, in association with other factors, lead to sphincter failure. Gastroesophageal incompetence also occurs as a consequence of disease or operations that destroy or bypass the intrinsic lower esophageal sphincter. Various other factors may contribute to gastroesophageal reflux and its complications, including overeating and obesity and their effect on intra-abdominal and intragastric pressures, gastric motility and gastric outlet patency and their effect on gastric emptying, and the physiologic effect of certain drugs and foods on the lower esophageal sphincter.

The complications of gastroesophageal reflux are shown in Table 1-1. Almost all of them are directly or indirectly related to the noxious effects of refluxed digestive secretions on the esophageal mucosa. Medical measures are aimed at minimizing the reflux, altering the corrosive effects of the refluxed secretions, enhancing gastric emptying and sphincter tone, and protecting the mucosa. These efforts are successful in most patients; however, in a few patients, progressive disabling complications persist despite all medical efforts. In a few patients who present for care, significant complications have already developed despite medical treatment. The patients in whom medical treatment fails are potential candidates for surgical treatment.

Surgical treatment is restricted to two basic endeavors: (1) restoration of gastroesophageal competence or (2) alteration of the corrosive quality of refluxed secretions. Restoration of competence is the more physiologic and more desirable of the two alternatives; however, under special circumstances (to be defined), the second alternative becomes most attractive. This discussion is not to decry the various other effective alternatives for reconstruction of the esophagus and esophagogastric continuity. The two approaches to be described are not only the extremes of the available operations but also two safe and effective solutions.

TABLE 1-1. Complications of gastroesophageal reflux

Complication
Intractable distress
Esophagitis
Bleeding
Stricture of esophagus
Reversible
Irreversible
Shortened esophagus
Esophageal perforation
Columnar epithelial-lined lower esophagus (Barrett's esophagus)
Motility disturbance of the esophagus
Contraction rings of the lower esophagus
Aspiration

Treatment Strategies

The chief goals of clinical investigation of a patient with gastroesophageal reflux are to define the complications that are present and to determine as clearly as possible those that are directly attributable to reflux and thereby reversible. In most patients, these goals can be achieved by means of a detailed clinical history supplemented by objective data obtained from radiographic examination, endoscopy, and manometric studies of esophageal motility. Only occasionally are such data insufficient to define the cause of a patient's subjective complaints. Thus, in the absence of objective esophageal aberration, one may have to resort to an acid reflux test, perform an esophageal bougienage to define the nature and pliability of apparent esophageal obstruction, or use videoradiography or cineradiography with or without the ingestion of solids mixed with contrast media.

After delineation of the extent of objective and subjective abnormalities, their potential for reversibility or progression must be assessed, especially if the patient has not attempted a vigorous medical program. Many subjective and objective reflux problems are amenable to a good medical program of weight reduction, a head-up bed, topical antacids, H-2 blockade of gastric secretion, abstinence from tobacco and alcohol, and the addition of agents such as metoclopramide, which enhance gastric emptying and the tone of the lower esophageal sphincter. When disabling subjective symptoms and objective reflux changes persist despite medical efforts, surgical intervention should be considered.

Various contingencies must be considered. If a stenosis is present in the esophagus, the main consideration is whether it is readily dilatable to a 50-F size or whether it is a tight stricture that will require resection for relief. In practice, almost all strictures can be successfully dilated to a 50-F size; for the few that cannot be dilated, special surgical efforts are required. Axiomatic for the dilatable stenosis secondary to reflux is the fact that it is permanently reversible if the noxious effects of reflux can be controlled.

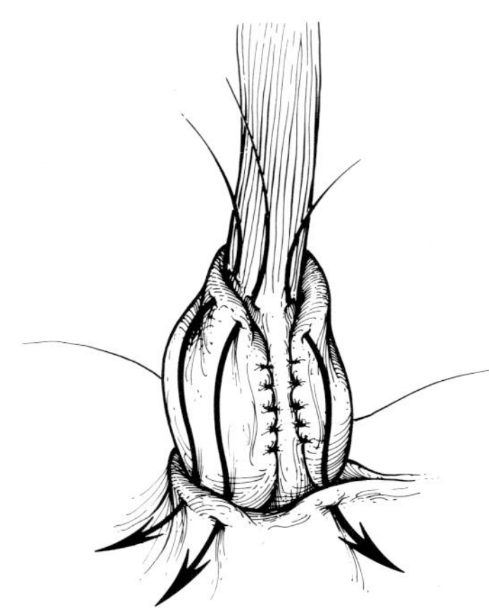

Uncut Collis
Gastroplasty
270° Fundoplication

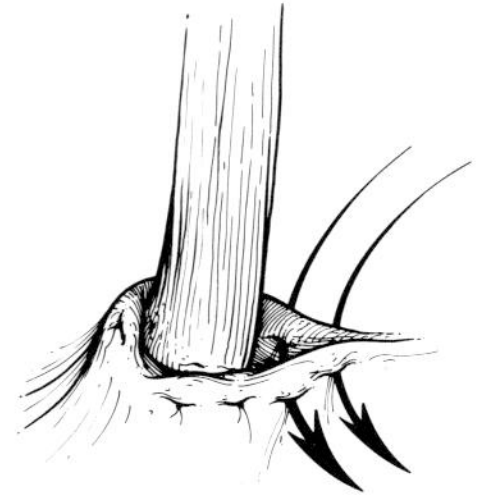

Final Reduction
Crural Repair
270° Fundoplication

A shortened esophagus poses another surgical dilemma. If the esophagus is found to be truly shortened at operation, standard reduction and repair of the hiatal hernia with antireflux measures is not possible. In practice, a truly shortened esophagus is rare; but when it is suspected, a transthoracic approach is required. If a shortened esophagus is present and is unrelieved by extensive distal esophageal mobilization, an esophageal lengthening procedure is necessary. This is usually effected by the performance of a Collis gastroplasty with one of the antireflux fundoplications. On occasion, even this procedure cannot be performed to advantage, and vagotomy-antrectomy-Roux-Y becomes a desirable alternative.

The presence or absence of esophageal peristalsis is another important consideration when an antireflux procedure is planned because the 360° fundoplications of the Nissen type are often too obstructive, even when loosely wrapped around an amotile esophagus. In such circumstances, one of the 270° fundoplications of the Belsey type should be considered.

Further, one should consider whether a gastric operation has been performed previously. Previous distal gastric resection may not have left a sufficient proximal gastric remnant to effect a fundoplication. Further, a previous gastric fundoplication may have permanently distorted the fundus so as to render it unsuitable for further fundoplication. Indeed, the present reflux problem may be secondary to a previous operation in which the proximal stomach and lower esophageal sphincter were removed. These problems can all be solved with the long-limb Roux-Y gastric drainage procedure. Fortunately, most patients with reflux problems have not had a previous gastric operation or hiatal hernia repair that could potentially preclude an antireflux procedure.

Finally, one must always question whether a previous operation or operations have left the vagal trunks intact. Ordinarily, vagotomy should not be part of an antireflux procedure; however, if it has been performed, it may have deleterious effects on gastric emptying unless accompanied by a gastric drainage procedure. The exception is the highly selective parietal cell vagotomy. In our experience, gastroesophageal reflux has, in some cases, disappeared after accidental vagotomy when gastric drainage was enhanced by performing pyloroplasty alone. Thus, for patients suspected of having gastroesophageal reflux, it is essential not only to establish reflux as the cause of the symptoms and to define complications in terms of their severity and reversibility but also to review in detail the specific factors that potentially contribute to the problem, including previously performed operations and preexisting esophageal or gastroduodenal disease. With such information, an intelligent and rational decision can be made regarding the need for and type of surgical intervention. In brief, the surgical strategies can be summarized as follows.

1. When reflux is associated with an esophageal hiatal hernia and objective complications are potentially reversible, an antireflux procedure is indicated. The author favors a left transthoracic, modified, uncut, 30-mm Collis gastroplasty with a 360° Nissen-type fundoplication. If esophageal motility is absent (as in scleroderma of the esophagus or postesophagomyotomy states), a 270° Belsey-type fundoplication is preferred.

2. When the esophagus is shortened (usually as a consequence of reflux esophagitis) and the stomach cannot be reduced below the diaphragm despite surgical mobilization, the author favors a cut, 55-mm Collis gastroplasty with fundoplication; again, the type of fundoplication is dictated by the presence or absence of esophageal peristalsis.

3. When gastroesophageal reflux is associated with an esophageal stenosis that cannot be dilated to 50-F size, resection of the esophageal stricture becomes mandatory. For a short, well-localized, undilatable stricture, a conservative esophageal resection with esophagogastrostomy is indicated. This procedure invariably results in complete vagotomy, loss of the lower esophageal sphincter, and an acquired shortening of the esophagus. The author favors transabdominal gastric antrectomy and an 18-inch Roux-Y gastric drainage procedure. This technique effectively alters the corrosive quality of the gastric contents. Such a gastric drainage procedure with antrectomy-vagotomy is also applicable for the rare circumstance in which transmural esophagitis has totally and permanently fixed the shortened esophagus in the mediastinum so that mobilization and antireflux measures are technically impossible to achieve. For long, undilatable esophageal strictures or for those located in the middle and upper thirds of the thoracic esophagus, a modified Ivor-Lewis-type resection and reconstruction is recommended. This can also be accomplished as a combined transcervical, transhiatal total esophagectomy without thoracotomy. In these circumstances, resection of the stomach is usually not necessary. The stomach is usually brought to the apex of the chest above the azygos vein or to the neck for esophagogastrostomy. If care is taken to perform a high anastomosis and ensure a totally intrathoracic stomach, late reflux problems are rare despite the sphincter loss and absence of esophagogastric valvuloplasty.

Surgical Technique

Modified (Uncut) Collis Gastroplasty With Fundoplication. The technique of left transthoracic, modified (uncut) Collis gastroplasty with a 360° Nissen fundoplication is the most common of the surgical alternatives to be discussed. The patient is positioned under general anesthesia in the right lateral decubitus position. After preparation and draping of the left thorax, a posterolateral thoracotomy is performed, and the left pleural space is entered through the bed of the nonresected left eighth rib (seventh intercostal space). The inferior pulmonary ligament is divided, and the lung is retracted cephalad. By blunt and sharp dissection, the distal esophagus is freed, and a large Penrose drain is passed around the lower esophagus and vagi to elevate these structures from the posterior mediastinum (Fig. 1-44).

At this point, if it was not apparent earlier, a sliding esophageal hiatal hernia is usually clearly definable, and several centimeters of stomach and the esophagogastric junction are displaced above the diaphragm through the esophageal hiatus into the chest. A peritoneal hernia sac covers the anterolateral aspect of this herniated stomach. An incision into this sac gives free access to the peritoneal cavity through the esophageal hiatus. A Richardson retractor is inserted through the hiatus, and traction is applied ventrally. The left hand of the surgeon is inserted through the patulous hiatus with the index finger on the thoracic side and the other three fingers on the abdominal side of the phrenoesophageal ligament medial to the esophagus. With the phrenoesophageal ligament and underlying peritoneum under traction, they are divided with scissors. The upper gastrohepatic omentum is clamped, divided, and ligated through the esophageal hiatus. Care is taken to identify and preserve the vagal trunks.

As the attachments between the esophagogastric junction and dia-

Figure 1-44

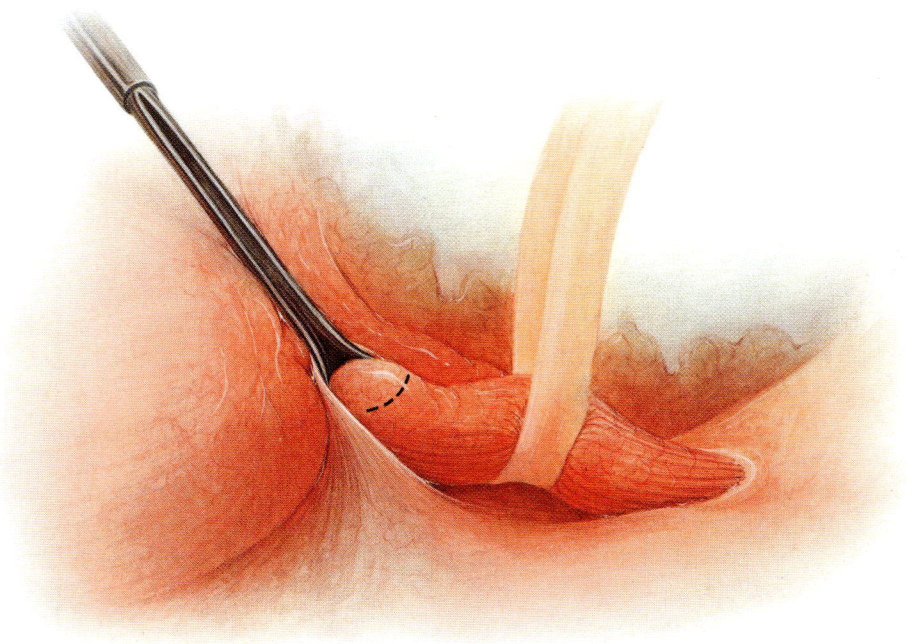

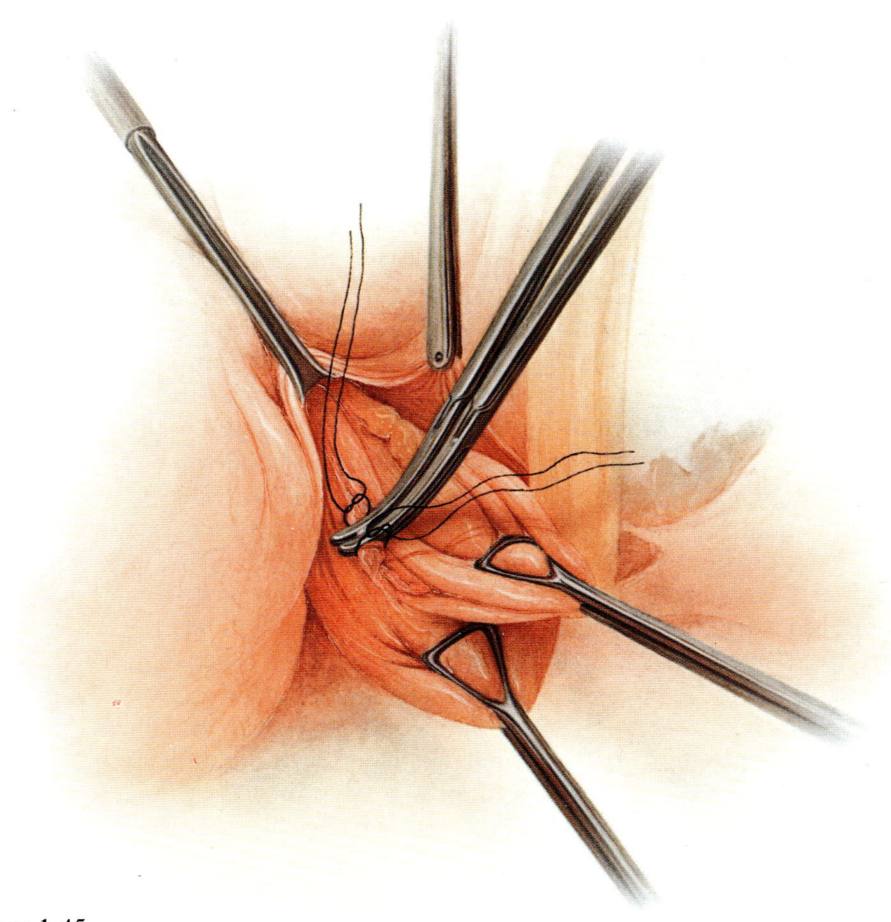

Figure 1-45

Figure 1-46

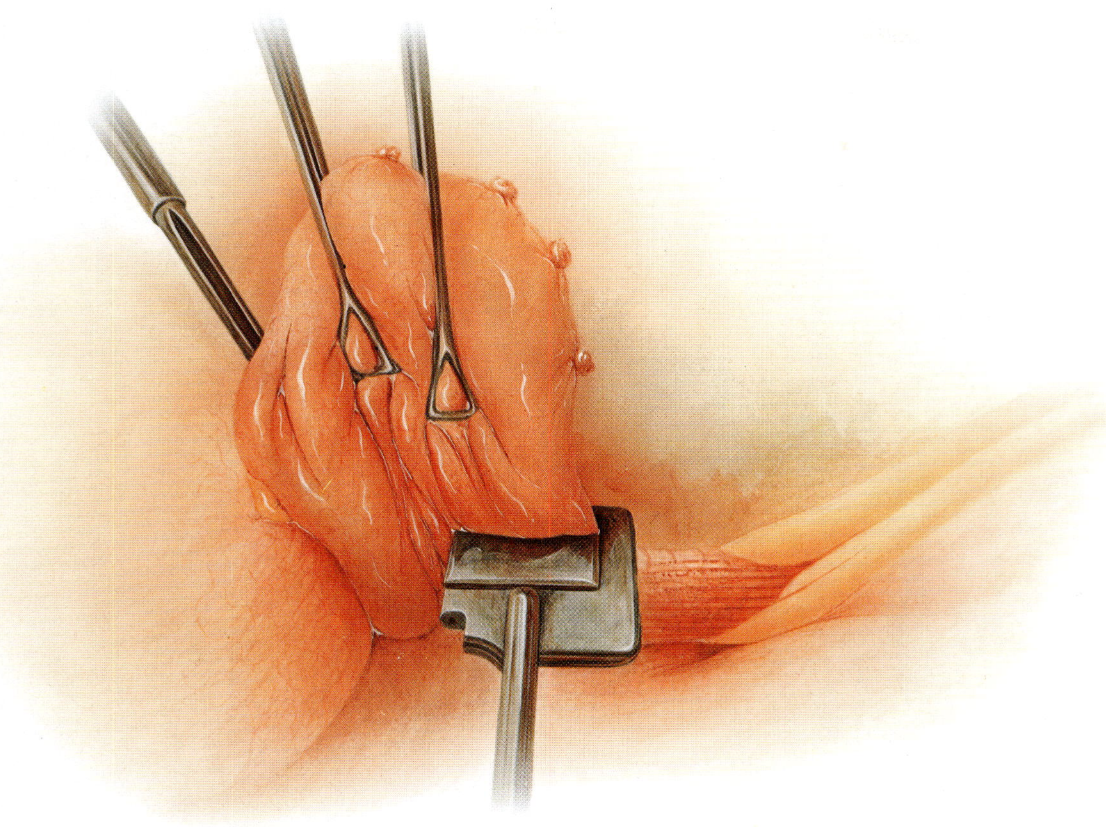

phragm are divided, more and more of the proximal stomach can be drawn into the thorax through the hiatus. The fundus and greater curvature of the stomach, however, are firmly anchored in the abdomen by short gastric vessels. By grasping the anterior aspect of the stomach with lung clamps (Fig. 1-45), these short gastric vessels can be exposed through the hiatus and individually clamped, divided, and ligated. In step fashion, the entire fundus and part of the upper greater curvature of the stomach are completely freed up to the esophagogastric junction (Fig. 1-46). With about 10 cm of the greater curvature of the stomach so mobilized into the chest, the esophagogastric fat pad is then excised. Again, care is taken to identify and preserve both vagal trunks. The passage of a 50-F Maloney dilator from the mouth down the esophagus into the stomach aids in this dissection.

Figure 1-47

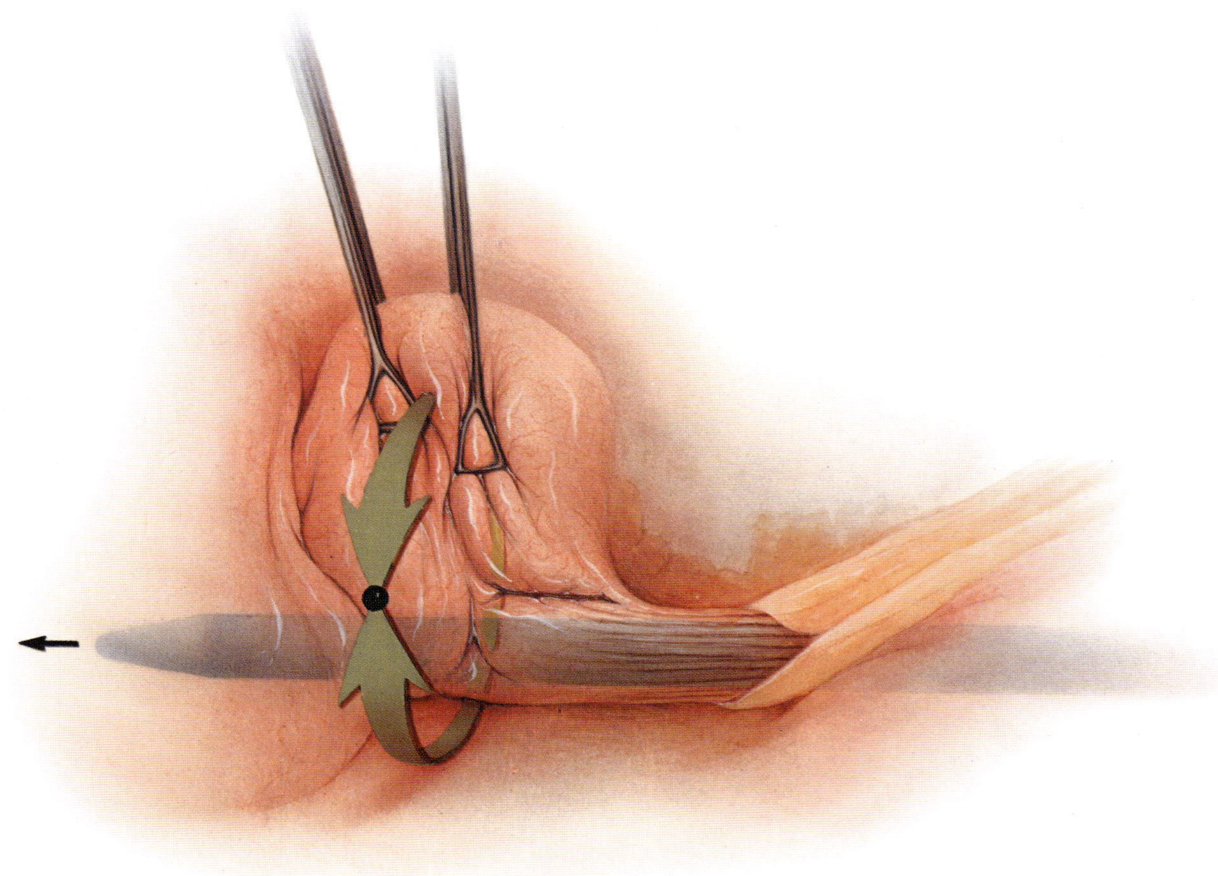

The greater curvature of the stomach is then grasped with lung clamps. With both the anterior and posterior aspects of the proximal stomach in clear view in the thorax, a TA 30 stapling device (without aligning pin) is applied to the stomach at the angle of His, parallel to the lesser curvature and the indwelling Maloney dilator (Fig. 1-46). The delivery of staples from this instrument creates an uncut tubular extension of the esophagus that is made up of the lesser curvature of the stomach (Fig. 1-47).

The fundus is then wrapped 360° around the neoesophagus. This fundoplication is anchored to the neoesophagus with multiple rows of interrupted 3-0 silk sutures (Fig. 1-48). This suture line and the staple line create a frenulum effect that prevents subsequent telescoping of the stomach out of the fundoplication (Fig. 1-49). Shown in cross section in Fig. 1-49 are vagal trunks that are wrapped with fundus and removed from potential suture injury.

Figure 1-48

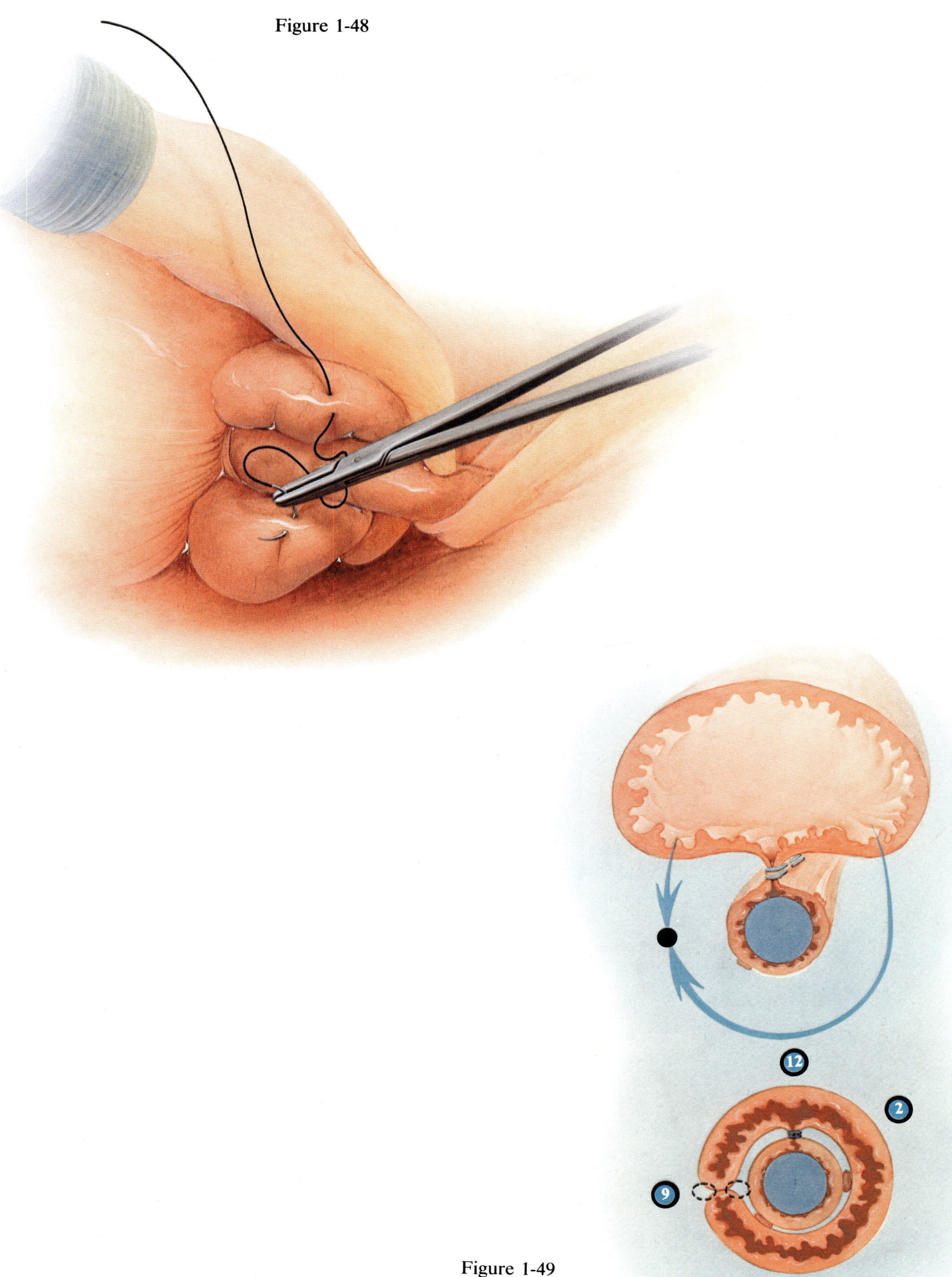

Figure 1-49

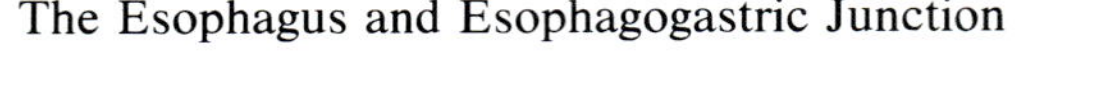

Figure 1-50

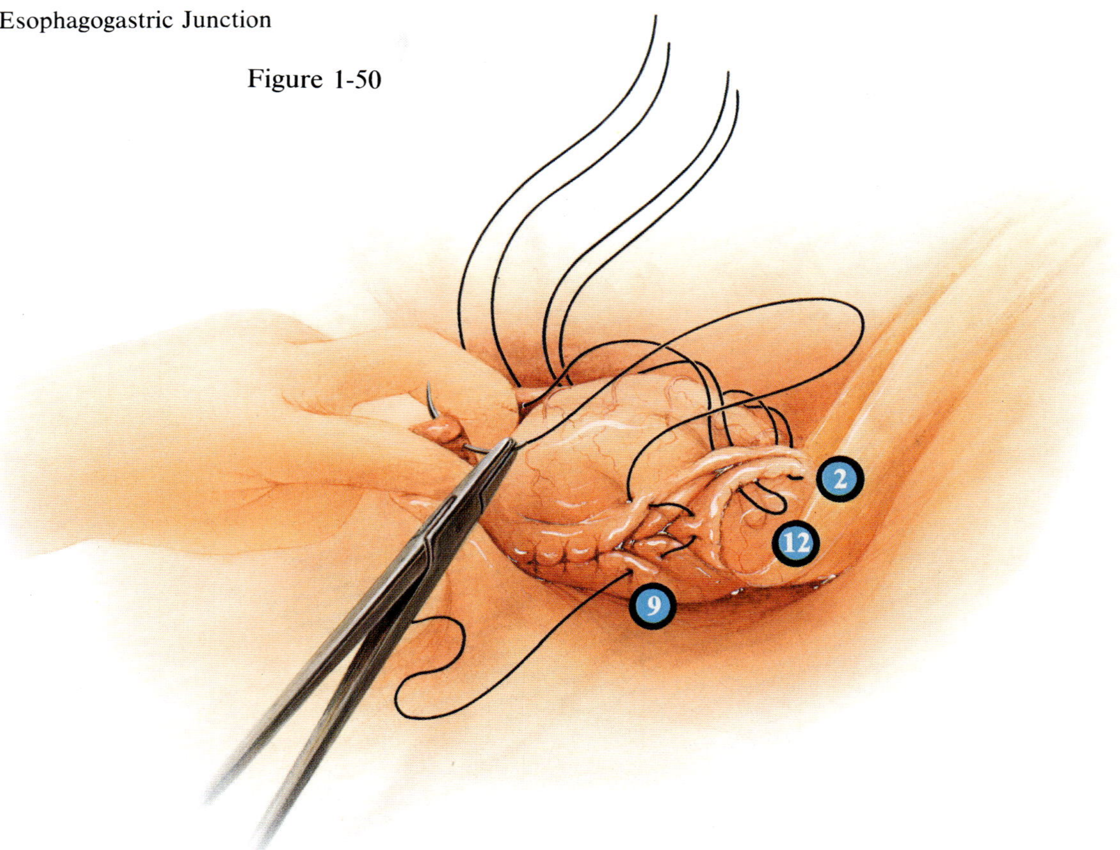

The entire fundoplication is then reduced below the diaphragm and anchored in place with three horizontal mattress sutures. They incorporate the remnants of the phrenoesophageal ligament and the upper edge of the fundus; they then pass through the esophageal hiatus and out the perihiatal diaphragm (Fig. 1-50). With reduction of the stomach and plication below the diaphragm, these sutures are tied to maintain reduction. In the cross-sectional drawing of Figure 1-49, note that these sutures are placed at the 9, 12, and 2 o'clock positions as viewed from above. Several crural stitches are placed behind the esophagus to create a snug, but not tight, hiatus (Fig. 1-51). With the 50-F Maloney dilator in place, the hiatus will admit one or two fingers with ease. The mediastinal pleura is closed, and the lung is reexpanded. The chest incision is closed, and a single catheter is brought from the left pleural space to the outside through a separate intercostal stab wound. A nasogastric tube is passed for postoperative suction drainage.

Intraoperative esophageal manometry before and after repair has shown that the procedure restores a high-pressure zone in the region of the fundoplication and gastroplasty. The length of the zone is related to the length of the gastroplasty and fundoplication.

270° Fundoplication. This partial fundoplication is used when esophageal peristalsis is proved to be absent with preoperative esophageal manometry. The reduction and repair are as described for the 360° fundoplication.

Cut Collis Gastroplasty. A GIA stapling device is applied to the stomach at the angle of His, parallel to the lesser curvature of the stomach and the

Figure 1-51

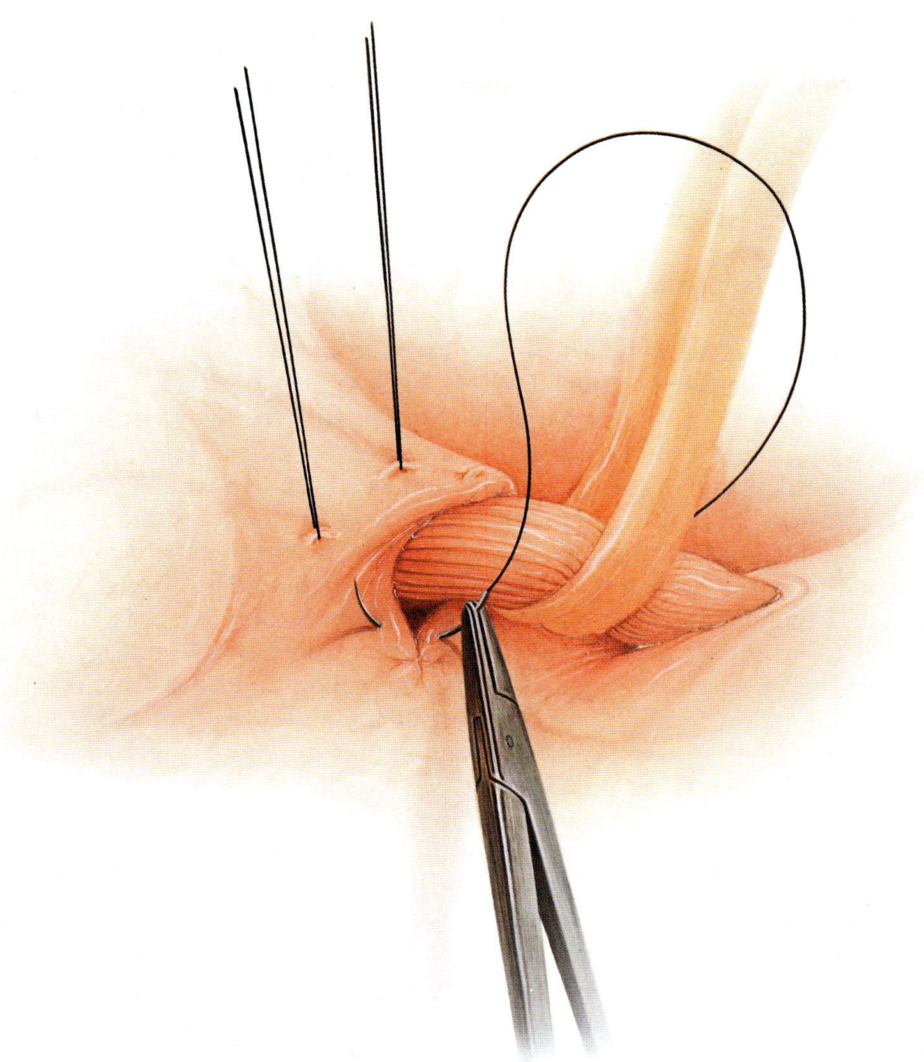

indwelling 50-F Maloney dilator. The advancement of the knife cuts and activates the delivery and crimping of rows of staples on either side of the incision. The rows of staples are then buried beneath a row of interrupted 3-0 silk sutures. A mattress suture at the very apex of the cut is placed to prevent tearing and bleeding at this unstapled, vulnerable angle. In patients with a shortened esophagus, the fundus of the stomach is often attenuated, and after the cut Collis gastroplasty is performed, often little more than a finger-like pedicle of fundus encircles the neoesophagus.

Vagotomy-Antrectomy Roux-Y. The individual steps of truncal vagotomy-gastric antrectomy and an 18-inch-long Roux-Y gastric drainage procedure are identical to those shown in a subsequent chapter (see Fig. 3-18 and 3-34) and in the preceding section dealing with construction of a long-limb Roux-Y after total gastrectomy (Fig. 1-33 through 1-43). The exposure for vagotomy and conservative resection of an esophageal stricture if required is best obtained through a left, seventh intercostal thoracotomy. The favored technique of reanastomosis is a two-layered suture anastomosis over a 50-F Maloney dilator, as previously illustrated. The esophagus is reanastomosed to the stomach at the site where the strictured esophagus is

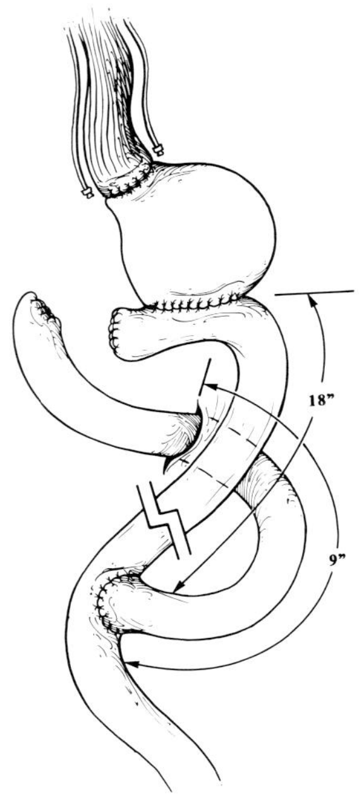

Vagotomy-Antrectomy
Roux-Y
Stricture Resection

disconnected from the stomach. Occasionally, the esophageal hiatus will need to be incised to mobilize the stomach into the chest; at other times, the best approach will actually be to close the cardia at the distal gastric site of esophageal resection and rotate the fundus into the chest for esophagogastrostomy. In patients without stricture or in whom the stricture is readily dilatable, distal esophageal resection is not required, and the only necessary step is either transthoracic or transabdominal vagotomy.

The distal gastric resection and construction of the long-limb Roux-Y gastric drainage procedure is best effected through an upper midline abdominal incision. The technical details of antrectomy are discussed in Chapter 3. The details of Roux-Y construction are reviewed in "Total Gastrectomy (Roux-Y)," this chapter. Basically, the Roux-Y procedure entails dividing the jejunum 9 inches (23 cm) from the ligament of Treitz and carrying the division deep into the mesentery of the jejunum at that point. The distal end of the divided jejunum is closed, a postcolic, antiperistaltic end-to-side gastrojejunostomy is performed in layers, and the remnant of stomach is anchored to the defect in the transverse mesocolon just above the gastrojejunostomy. The end-to-side jejunojejunostomy is performed 18 inches (46 cm) distal to the gastrojejunostomy. Care is taken to close all intersecting mesenteries to prevent internal herniation (Fig. 1-43). This procedure of suppression of gastric secretion and biliary-pancreatic diversion is less desirable than those procedures that restore competence to the cardia. Gastroesophageal reflux continues, but it is bland and innocuous because the gastric contents have been altered so that they do not contain acid, bile, or pancreatic secretions. Preexisting respiratory aspiration is a relative contraindication; if it is present prior to operation, it is likely to persist after this procedure. Further, an additional, although low, risk is the development of dumping and diarrhea and diminished gastric reservoir capacity with attendant weight loss. Despite these potential disadvantages, in most selected patients in whom vagotomy-antrectomy Roux-Y is performed, it is often the only alternative or most dependable of the available options. It should be further emphasized that complete vagotomy is essential for success. Incomplete vagotomy is associated with persistent acid secretion, persistent corrosive esophagitis, and the occurrence of marginal ulceration at the gastrojejunostomy. The Roux-Y configuration of the gastric drainage procedure is not essential, but the length of bowel between the gastrojejunostomy and the biliary-pancreatic secretions is essential. Failure to construct a sufficiently long segment (minimum of 18 inches) is to risk not only bile esophagitis but also bile gastritis.

Postoperative Care

The care of patients who undergo antireflux procedures is similar to that of patients who undergo any type of thoracotomy. The care of patients who undergo vagotomy, antrectomy, and a Roux-Y gastric drainage procedure differs little from that of patients who undergo any other transabdominal gastric operation. The one exception is our compulsion to perform a Gastrografin contrast study on all patients who have undergone an esophageal operation prior to instituting an oral diet. If leakage is encountered, a subclavian venous parenteral alimentation line is inserted, and oral intake is withheld until sufficient healing occurs. The details of this approach are described on page 20. In most patients, the Gastrografin study will indicate normal patency of the anastomoses without extravasation. In these cases, oral intake can generally be resumed the day after operation and can rapidly progress during the ensuing 3 to 4 days to a general diet. The chest tubes and nasogastric tube are generally removed the day after operation, and the patient is urged to begin showering and shampooing early during the postoperative stage. Hospital dismissal is usually feasible within a week of operation.

Results

The antireflux procedures described have been most effective—less than 5% of patients experience recurrent disease. Anatomic hernia recurrence, telescoped fundoplication, gas-bloat syndrome, or concomitant splenectomy and operative death have been virtually absent. Despite these advantages, morbidity has been notable. About 5% of patients have experienced annoying dysphagia without apparent or definable cause. Leakage from suture or staple lines has occurred infrequently; when this complication is detected by Gastrografin study and managed as described, it rarely poses a serious threat. Despite these shortcomings, 90% of patients have a highly satisfactory long-term result.

Patients who undergo resecting and diverting procedures to prevent the corrosive effects of gastroesophageal reflux have had a higher risk of complications. The operative mortality has been 1%, and the incidence of digestive distress directly attributable to vagotomy or gastric resection has been 10%. Esophagitis and its complications have been gratifyingly controlled in virtually all patients.

Achalasia

Achalasia is the most common of the specific motility disturbances of the esophagus. It is an acquired condition that affects persons from childhood through old age. Although the precise inciting factors are unknown, the condition is known to be due to degeneration of vagal innervation of the thoracic esophagus and its lower esophageal sphincter. The consequences of this decreased parasympathetic innervation are the loss of coordinated sequential or peristaltic contractions in the body of the esophagus and the failure of appropriate relaxation of the lower esophageal sphincter with swallowing.

The clinical symptoms that develop as a consequence of these functional disturbances are esophageal obstruction, retention, and regurgitation. Thus, patients complain of variable and unpredictable dysphagia or obstruction to the passage of swallowed solids or liquids. Additionally, because emptying of the esophagus into the stomach is partial or incomplete, pressure sensations in the retrosternal area may occur consequent to esophageal distention from retention. Some persons, especially those in whom achalasia is associated with vigorous simultaneous nonperistaltic contractions in the body of the esophagus, may have episodic pain that is indistinguishable from that of acute myocardial ischemia or dissecting thoracic aneurysm. Esophageal retention and stasis may evoke subjective heartburn and even inflammation and ulceration in the distal esophagus that are clinically and morphologically indistinguishable from those of gastroesophageal reflux.

Despite an intact pharyngeal mechanism and a normal upper esophageal sphincter, spontaneous and postural regurgitation of esophageal contents into the pharynx, mouth, or nose frequently occurs. This material is characteristically bland, undigested, "fresh" food that is retained in the esophagus. Some patients may have retention and regurgitation of recently, insensibly swallowed saliva that is regurgitated as copious, thick mucus. Respiratory aspiration is an expected consequence of regurgitation, and this can eventually result in serious, irreversible injury to the lower respiratory tract.

Obstructions to swallowing in patients with achalasia can have serious effects on nutrition, growth, and development. Thus, some weight loss is not unusual. Most patients experience a weight loss of 10 to 40 lb (5 to 18 kg) when the condition is first diagnosed. Arrested growth and development, although potentially reversible with treatment, may be a striking feature in children and adolescents.

Finally, the worst complication of achalasia is the late development of esophageal malignant disease. This condition seems to occur most frequently in patients with long-standing (15 to 20 years) untreated or unrelieved achalasia. The tumors are epithelial cancers that may develop at any level in the esophagus and are rarely operable when diagnosed because the symptoms are often indistinguishable from those of chronic achalasia.

Diagnosis

Achalasia can be suspected with considerable accuracy on the basis of the clinical history. Fluoroscopic examination of the esophagus with ingested contrast medium will detect most cases of achalasia. The classic findings are a dilated, tortuous proximal esophagus with a tapered narrowing at the esophagogastric junction. About a third of patients will have a normal-caliber esophagus. However, esophageal manometry is the most definitive means of diagnosis. Esophageal endoscopy should also be performed at the time of diagnosis to rule out malignant disease and to define other associated or complicating factors, such as an epiphrenic diverticulum or esophageal hiatal hernia.

Treatment

The treatment of achalasia of the esophagus is entirely palliative. A "cure" for achalasia in the sense of restoring peristalsis and coordinated relaxation of the lower esophageal sphincter with swallowing has not been possible. The basic principle of current therapy is palliation by weakening the nonrelaxing lower esophageal sphincter to prevent obstruction and retention, but not to the extent that gastroesophageal reflux will occur. The goal of such treatment is long-term, subjective patient satisfaction. Qualitative changes in the results of esophageal motility studies are not expected, and megaesophagus, if present prior to treatment, remains essentially unchanged. Esophageal retention should be greatly diminished by treatment, and both the length and the magnitude of the high-pressure zone at the lower esophageal sphincter are diminished but not absent. Achalasia of the esophagus is not the same as Hirschsprung's disease of the colon, although both are due to parasympathetic denervation. In achalasia, both the obstructing, narrowed distal sphincteric area and the more proximal dilated portion exhibit denervation; but in Hirschsprung's disease, only the distal obstructing portion is without innervation. Thus, in achalasia, the proximal esophageal hypertrophy and dilatation are as much a part of the denervation process as is the distal narrowed segment and are not reversed when distal obstruction is relieved.

Figure 1-52

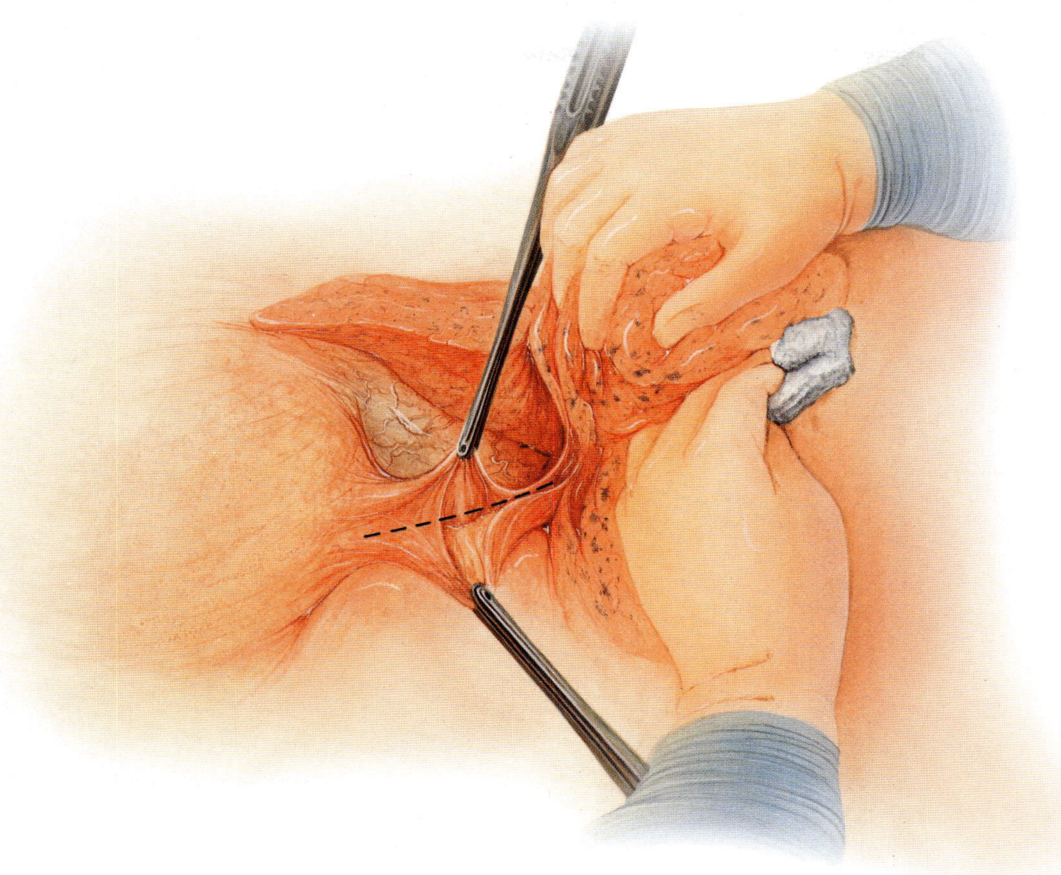

Two methods are used for relief of the distally obstructing, nonrelaxing lower esophageal sphincter: either forceful pneumatic or hydrostatic esophageal dilatation or surgical division by means of an extramucosal esophagomyotomy. Today, the surgical procedure has largely replaced dilatation because it provides significantly superior results. Persistent or recurrent attempts at forceful dilatation may result in hemorrhage and fibrosis in the esophageal wall, which can preclude the performance of an effective operation by fusing the dissection plane between the esophageal muscularis and mucosa.

Technique. A left thoracotomy provides exposure. The pleural space is entered through the bed of the unresected eighth rib. The inferior pulmonary ligament is divided, and the lung is retracted cephalad. The dome of the left diaphragm is retracted caudad. The divided mediastinal pleura is reflected anteriorly and posteriorly to expose the distal esophagus in the posterior mediastinum (Fig. 1-52). By blunt dissection, a broad Penrose drain is manually passed around the distal esophagus and adjacent vagal trunks to elevate them from the mediastinum (Fig. 1-53). Unusual distal traction on the esophagus is avoided to prevent drawing the stomach into the chest through the hiatus. With a scalpel, a vertical extramucosal myotomy is performed over a short distance (Fig. 1-54). A blunt-nosed, right-angled clamp is inserted through the myotomy to develop a dissection plane proximally and distally between the mucosa and muscularis

Figure 1-53

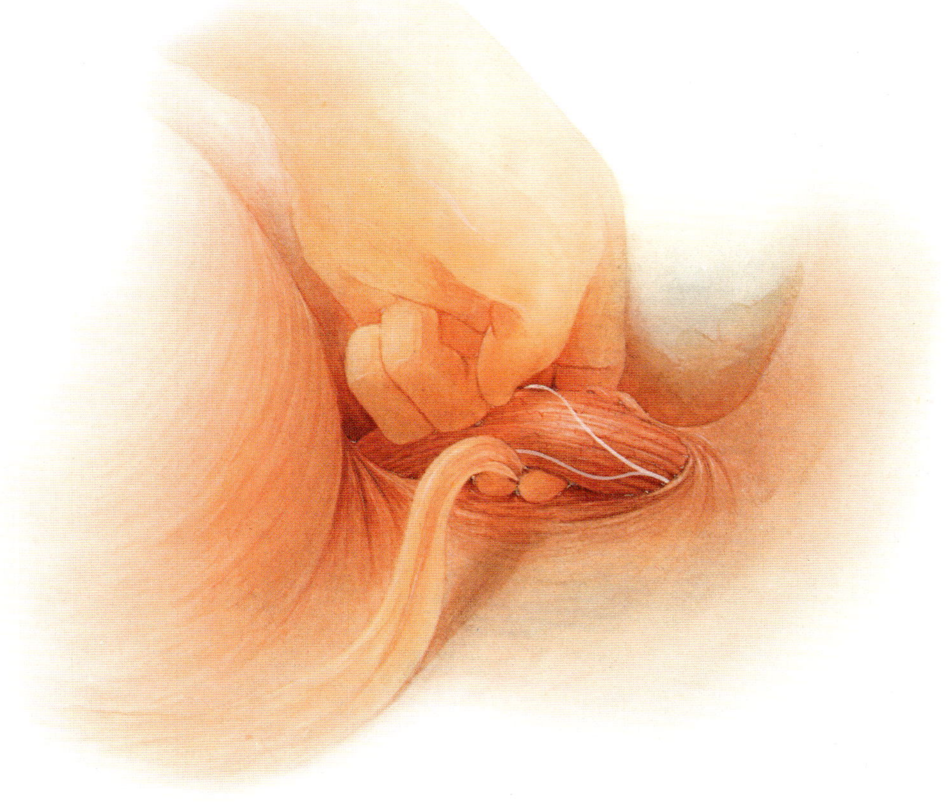

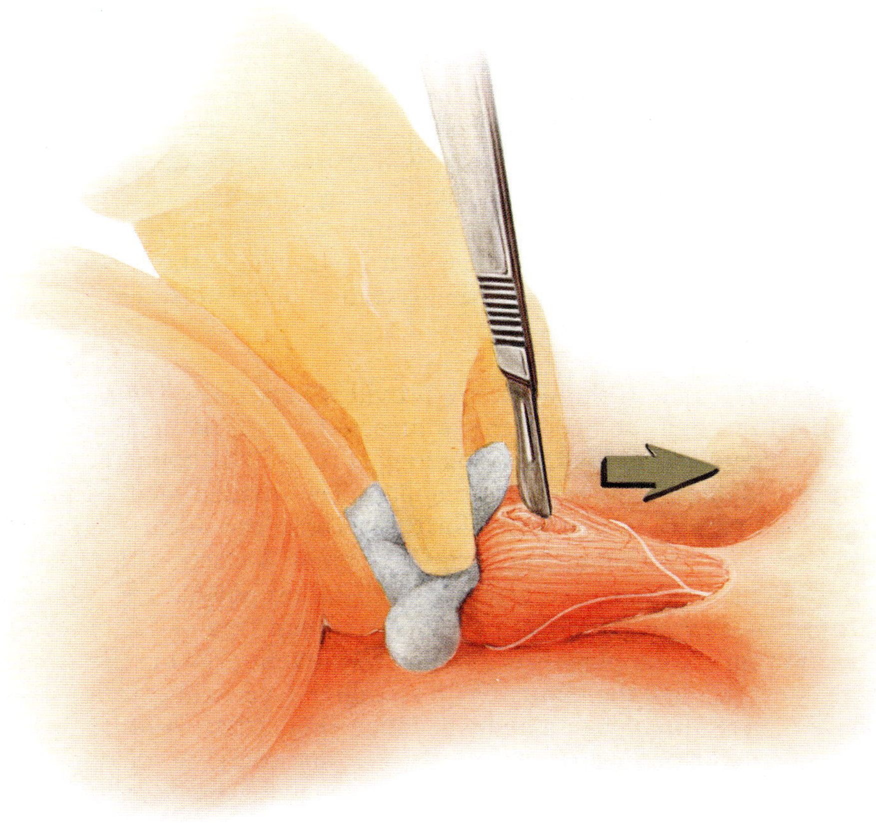

Figure 1-54

Figure 1-55

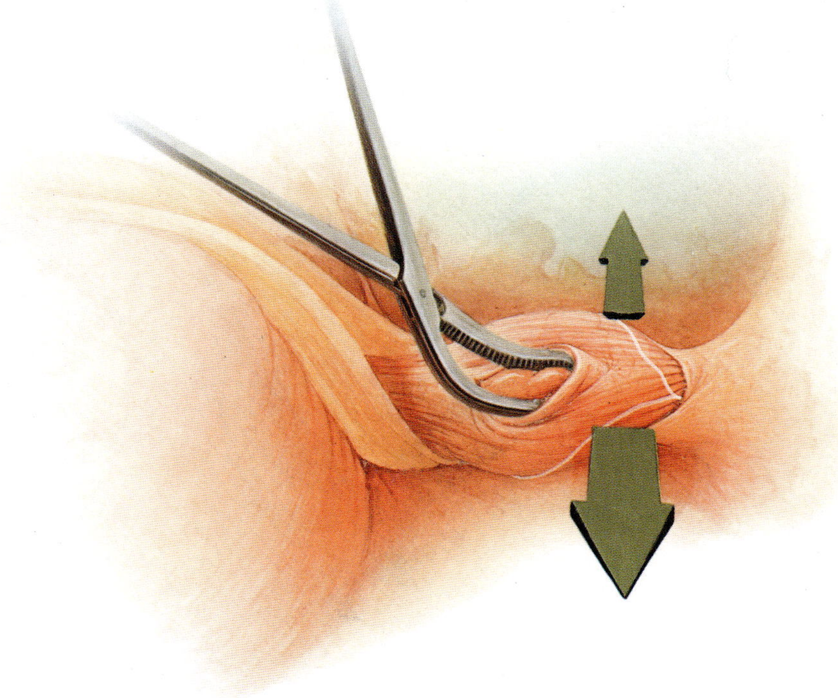

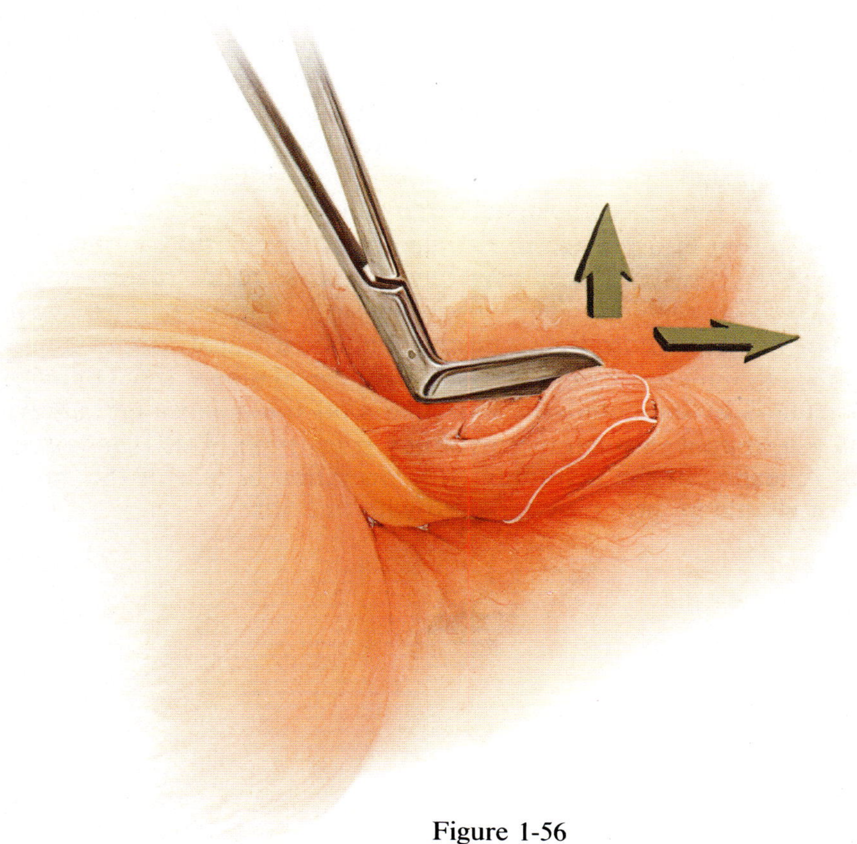

Figure 1-56

Figure 1-57

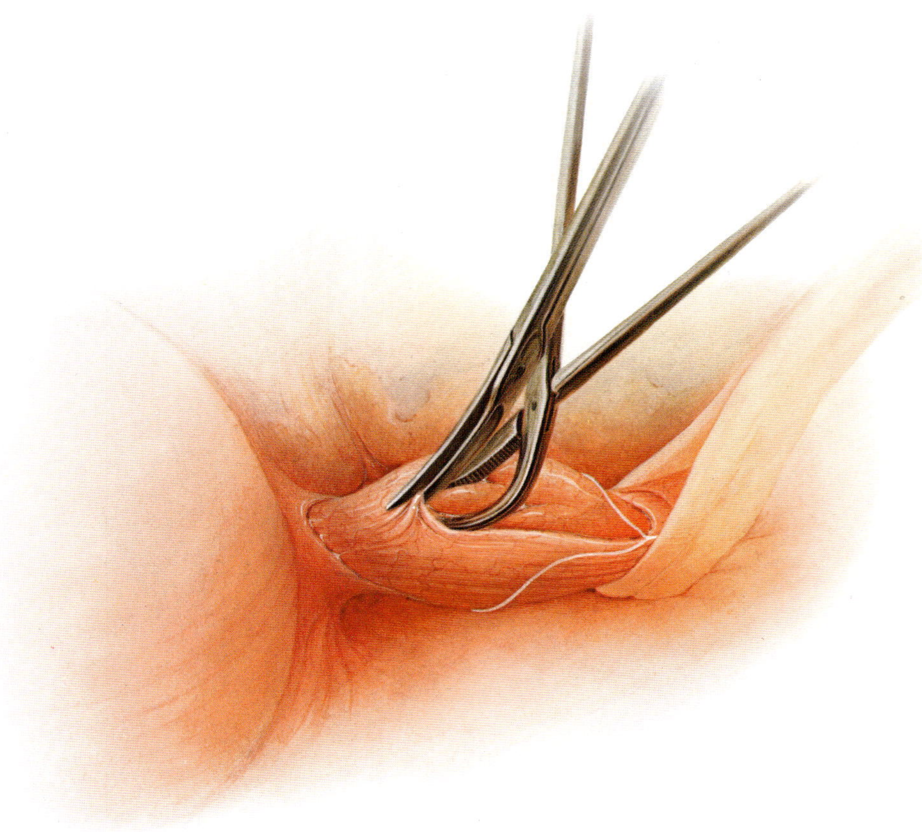

(Fig. 1-55). Myotomy is then readily extended proximally and distally from this point by either scalpel or scissors (Fig. 1-56 and 1-57). The author has modified a bandage scissors for this purpose (Fig. 1-56). The myotomy is extended proximally to the level of the inferior pulmonary vein in this manner. Distally, scalpel dissection is favored for the final few distal centimeters of esophagomyotomy because this is the critical part of the operation (Fig. 1-58). Basically, the distal extension of the myotomy depends on the identification of a change in extramucosal vascularity as one passes from the sparsely vascularized esophageal mucosa to the highly vascular rete of vessels characteristic of gastric mucosa. Extension of the myotomy more than 4 to 5 mm onto the stomach should be avoided. Approximately 50% of the circumference of the esophagel mucosal tube is freed of overlying muscularis by dissecting the muscularis off the mucosa and allowing the mucosa to pout through the myotomy (Fig. 1-59). This is required to prevent rehealing of the myotomy. If a laceration or tear of the mucosa occurs, it should be promptly repaired with fine silk.

Figure 1-58

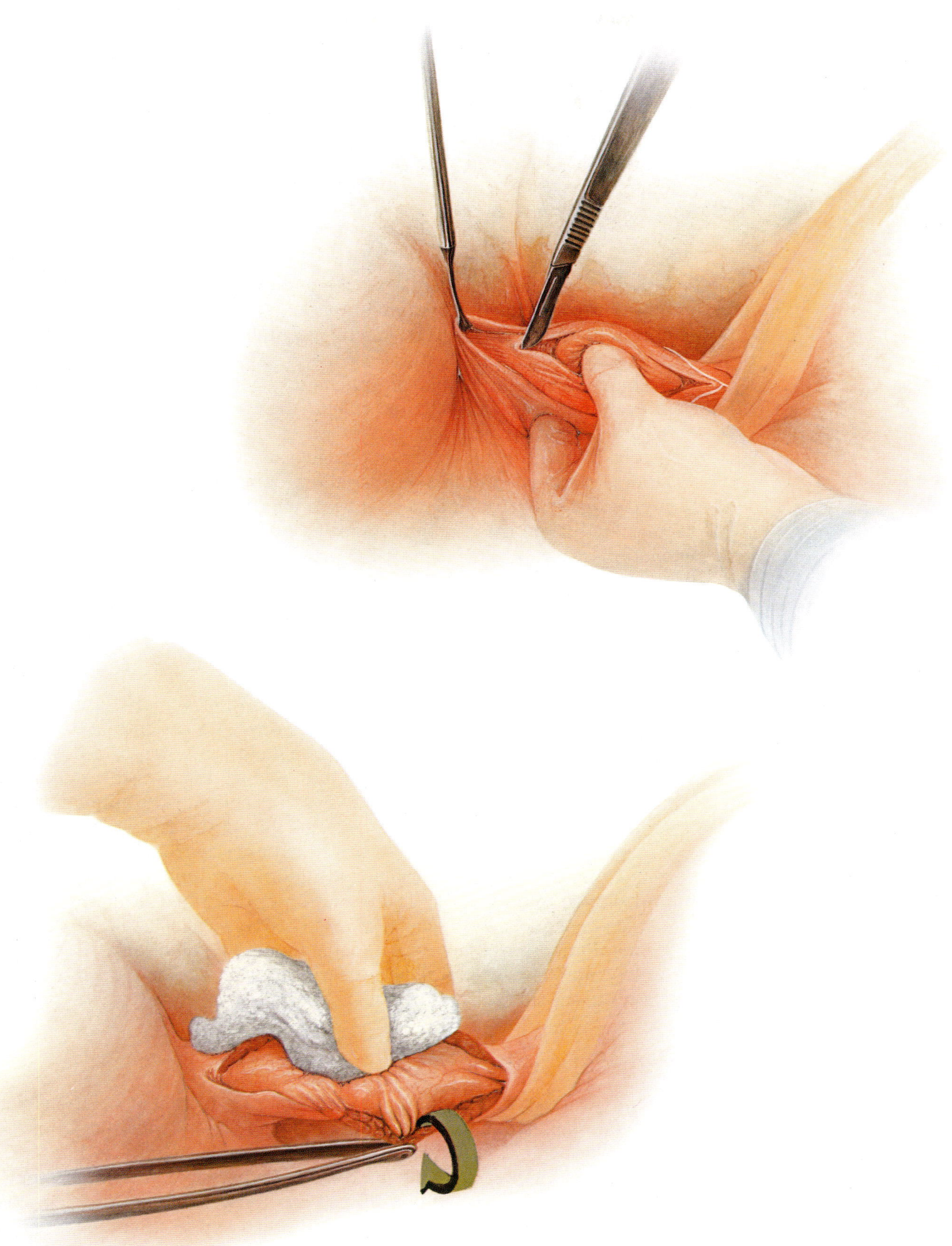

Figure 1-59

The esophagus is returned to its mediastinal bed, the mediastinal pleura is approximated loosely, the lung is reexpanded, the chest is closed, and a single catheter for postoperative suction drainage is brought from the left pleural space to the outside through a stab wound. A nasogastric tube is inserted prior to closure of the chest.

In recent years, we have found it helpful to perform intraoperative esophageal manometry before and after myotomy to ensure that a significant reduction in the length and magnitude of the distal esophageal high-pressure zone has been effected and that a portion of the infrahiatal sphincter persists. Even though such steps ensure effective division at the time of operation, they do not always guarantee a long-term satisfactory result.

Postoperative Care. Patients who undergo transthoracic esophagomyotomy are managed the same as patients who undergo any thoracic exploration. Analgesia, fluid replacement, vital signs, urinary output, and chest drainage are carefully monitored. Nasogastric tube suction drainage is continued overnight. On the morning after operation, a chest roentgenogram is obtained and fluoroscopic examination of the esophagus with water-soluble contrast media is performed. If no evidence of esophageal leakage is found, the chest tube and nasogastric tube are removed and an oral diet is resumed, and this diet rapidly progresses from liquids to solids during the next 48 to 72 hours. Intravenous administration of fluids is discontinued when the oral intake is sufficient. Chest roentgenography is repeated. Ambulation is begun the day after operation. Most patients are dismissed in 7 days. They are advised to restrict their activities and to avoid vigorous physical activities for approximately 6 weeks. Showering is begun early during the postoperative course, and most patients are able to walk several miles per day shortly after dismissal.

Results. The operative procedure described is extremely safe; in our experience, only one death occurred in 400 operated patients. Essentially all patients experience immediate and complete remission of all esophageal symptoms after operation. Such favorable results persist for decades in most patients, but approximately 15% will experience the gradual return of some or all of their previous symptoms during the ensuing months or years. Gastroesophageal reflux is rare. In our experience with 400 patients who had long-term follow-up, major symptoms or complications from reflux developed in only 2.5%. The operation as described is more likely to fail as a consequence of recurrent obstructive achalasia than of reflux problems. Patients who are experiencing favorable palliation at 1 year are extremely unlikely to experience deterioration in subjective esophageal function during subsequent decades.

Historical Comment

Over the years, surgeons have devised various technical solutions for benign and malignant conditions of the esophagogastric junction. Some of the better-known but largely discarded procedures are shown in Fig. 1-60. All of these techniques are associated with a higher incidence of poor long-term functional results than are current methods. The chief problem has been a high incidence of gastroesophageal reflux and its attendant complications of heartburn, esophagitis, and stricture formation when the lower

Achalasia

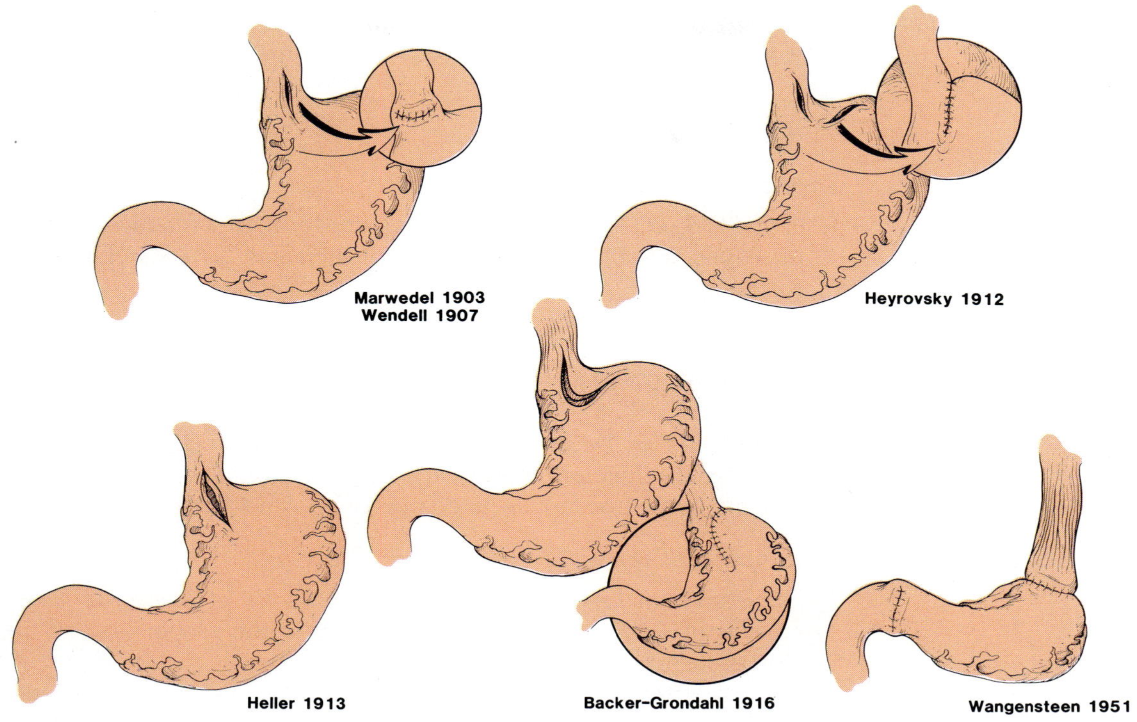

Esophagogastrectomy

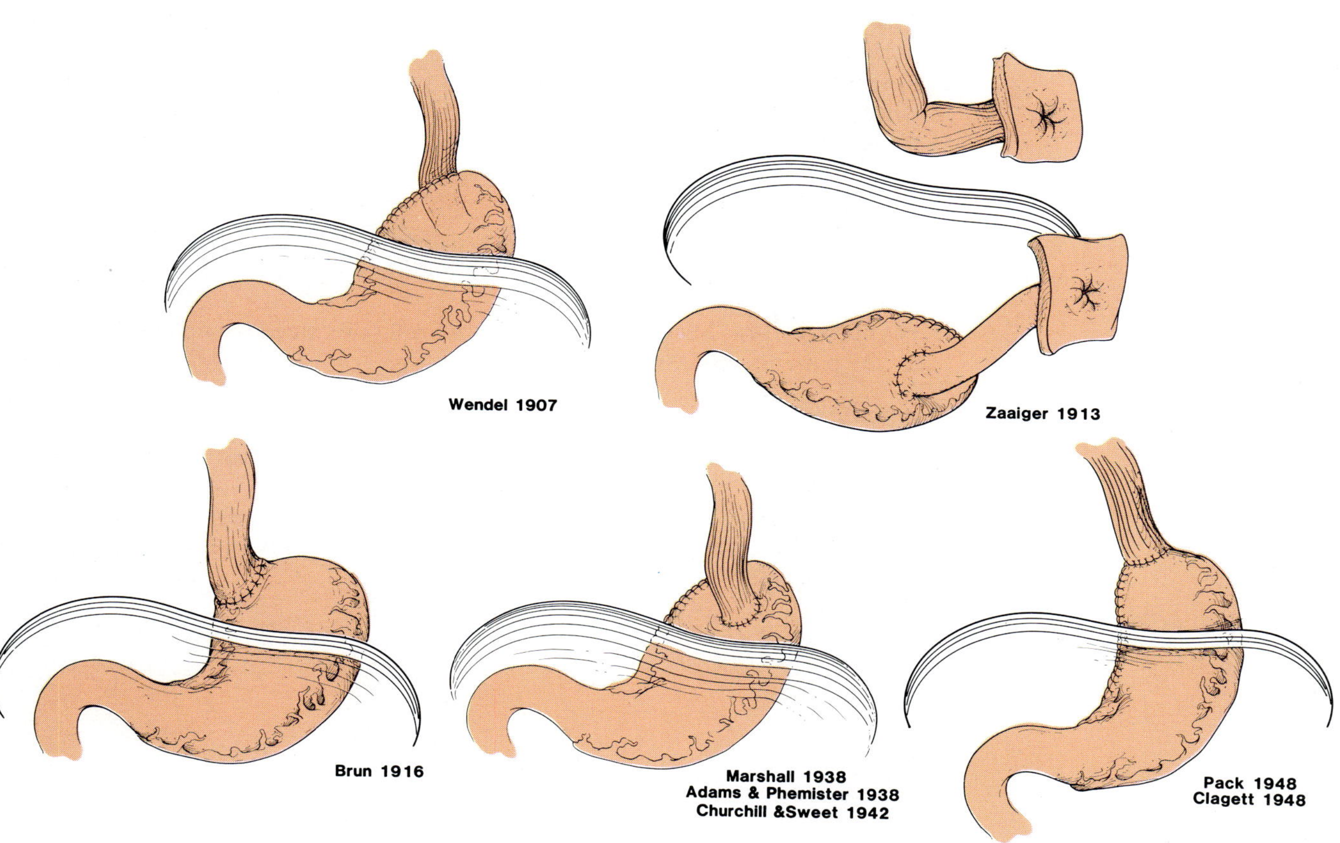

Figure 1-60

esophageal sphincter has been completely destroyed, bypassed, or resected. Many patients who have undergone these procedures and had bad results have been effectively salvaged with the gastric antrectomy with long-limb Roux-Y gastric drainage procedure (pages 49 and 50).

Suggested Reading

Surgical Anatomy

1. Payne WS, Olsen AM (1974) The origin, form, and function of the esophagus. In: Payne WS, Olsen AM (eds): The esophagus. Lea & Febiger, Philadelphia, p 1

Physiology

1. Goyal RK (1976) The lower esophageal sphincter. Viewpoints Dig Dis (December) 8, no. 3
2. O'Sullivan GC, DeMeester TR, Joelsson BE, et al (1982) Interaction of lower esophageal sphincter pressure and length of sphincter in the abdomen as determinants of gastroesophageal competence. Am J Surg 143: 40

Carcinoma of the Esophagogastric Junction

1. Gunnlaugsson GH, Wychulis AR, Roland C, et al (1970) Analysis of the records of 1,657 patients with carcinoma of the esophagus and cardia of the stomach. Surg Gynecol Obstet 130: 997
2. Lewis I (1946) The surgical treatment of carcinoma of the oesophagus: with special reference to a new operation for growths of the middle third. Br J Surg 34: 18
3. Payne WS (1972) The long-term clinical state after resection with total gastrectomy and Roux loop anastomosis. In: Smith RA, Smith RE (eds) Surgery of the oesophagus: the Coventry Conference. Appleton-Century-Crofts, New York, p 23
4. Payne WS, Bernatz PE (1976) One-stage resection and reconstruction for carcinoma of the esophagogastric junction. In: Varco RL, Delaney JP (eds) Controversy in surgery. WB Saunders, Philadelphia, p 593

Gastroesophageal Reflux and Its Complications

1. Piehler JM, Payne WS, Cameron AJ, et al (1984) The uncut Collis-Nissen procedure for esophageal hiatal hernia and its complications. Probl Gen Surg 1: 1
2. Payne WS (1984) Surgical management of reflux-induced oesophageal stenoses in 101 patients. Br J Surg 71: 971

Achalasia

1. Ellis FH Jr, Olsen AM (1969) Achalasia of the esophagus. Major Probl Clin Surg 9: 1
2. Okike N, Payne WS, Neufeld DM, et al (1979) Esophagomyotomy versus forceful dilation for achalasia of the esophagus: results in 899 patients. Ann Thorac Surg 28: 119

Surgical Anatomy and Physiology of the Stomach

2

Jon A. van Heerden

Surgical Anatomy

The stomach, which is roughly "J" shaped, stretches from the esophagogastric junction to the pylorus. The pylorus is a definite musculofibrotic sphincter also known as the muscle of Torkildson. The stomach is divided into the following anatomic sections: (1) the fundus is the area superior to and to the left of the esophagogastric junction; (2) the body, the largest part of the stomach, is interposed between the fundus and the gastric antrum; (3) the antrum, the distal portion of the stomach, extends roughly from the gastric angularis to the pylorus; a tongue of gastric antrum extends higher proximally on the lesser curvature of the stomach; and (4) the cardia is a zone approximately 3 cm wide distal to the esophagogastric junction.

Peritoneal folds extend in a fanlike fashion from the lesser and greater curvatures to form the gastrohepatic and gastrocolic omenta, respectively. The stomach forms the principal anterior boundary of the lesser sac in conjunction with these two omenta.

The stomach has four distinct linings: (1) the serous or peritoneal coat; (2) the muscular coat, which is a combination of circular, longitudinal, and oblique fibers; (3) the submucous coat; and (4) the gastric mucosa, of which the muscularis mucosa is the innermost layer.

Blood Supply

Arterial (*Fig. 2-1*). The blood supply to the stomach is extremely rich. Total compromise of the blood supply is extremely difficult, as evidenced by purposeful devascularization procedures such as those used for the treatment of esophagogastric varices (Sugiura procedure). This abundant arterial supply arises primarily from the celiac axis and is divided into (1) the left gastric artery, which arises directly from the celiac axis and courses distally along the upper part of the lesser curvature; (2) the right gastric artery, which arises from either the common hepatic or the gastroduodenal artery and courses proximally along the lesser curvature to inosculate with the left gastric artery; (3) the right gastroepiploic artery, which usually arises from the gastroduodenal artery and courses proximally along the greater curvature; and (4) the left gastroepiploic artery, which, after arising from the distal splenic artery, courses distally along the greater curvature.

The gastroduodenal artery, which arises from the common hepatic artery, lies immediately posterior to the first portion of the duodenum. It terminates as the superior pancreatoduodenal artery, which, in turn, freely anastomoses with the inferior pancreatoduodenal artery, which arises from the superior mesenteric artery. This rich anastomosis and the anatomic location of the gastroduodenal artery give rise to the bleeding, at times catastrophic, when a posterior duodenal ulcer penetrates. Along the greater curvature, the point at which the branches of the right gastroepiploic vessels entering the gastric serosa change their direction is the approximate proximal border of the gastric antrum, which is usually immediately opposite the gastric angularis on the lesser curvature.

Venous. The veins of the stomach accompany the respective arteries and include (1) the left gastric or coronary vein, (2) the right gastric or pyloric vein, (3) the right gastroepiploic vein, and (4) the left gastroepiploic vein. The left and right gastric veins empty directly into the portal vein. The venous drainage of these two vessels is of absolute importance in portal hypertension. The distal esophageal veins (potential esophageal varices) anastomose freely with the left gastric vein.

Lymphatic Drainage

The lymphatic drainage of the stomach is conveniently divided into five groups: (1) the left gastric nodes, which accompany the left gastric artery and can, in turn, be further subdivided into upper, lower, and pericardial; (2) the right gastroepiploic nodes, which drain the distal half of the greater curvature of the stomach; (3) the pyloric nodes (subpyloric nodes); (4) the hepatic nodes, which are intimately related to the hepatic artery and to the common bile duct; and (5) the splenic hilar nodes, which are in the hilus of the spleen and drain the proximal half of the greater curvature, the fundus of the stomach, and the esophagogastric junction.

Nerve Supply (*Fig. 2-2*)

The nerve supply to the stomach is both sympathetic and parasympathetic. The sympathetic supply to the stomach arises mainly from the celiac and left phrenic plexuses. The parasympathetic supply is from the 10th cranial (vagus) nerve. The anterior portion of the stomach obtains its parasympathetic supply from one or two vagal trunks (left vagus nerve). Arising from the left vagus nerve, 1 to 3 cm above the esophagogastric junction, is the hepatic branch. The posterior portion of the stomach is supplied mainly by the right branch of the vagus nerve (posterior vagal trunk). The celiac branch of the vagus nerve arises from the posterior vagal trunk. Both the anterior and the posterior branches continue distally in the gastrohepatic omentum as the nerves of Latarjet. They terminate by supplying the antrum and pylorus in an anatomic fanlike arrangement, commonly known as the "crow's foot."

The anterior vagus nerve (or nerves) is intimately related and applied to the surface of the esophagus and, in fact, may be somewhat embedded therein. In contrast, the posterior vagus nerve is clearly separate from the esophagus by a distance that might be 1 to 2 cm. In relation to the esophagus, the anterior and posterior trunks are roughly at the 11 and 7 o'clock positions, respectively.

Figure 2-1

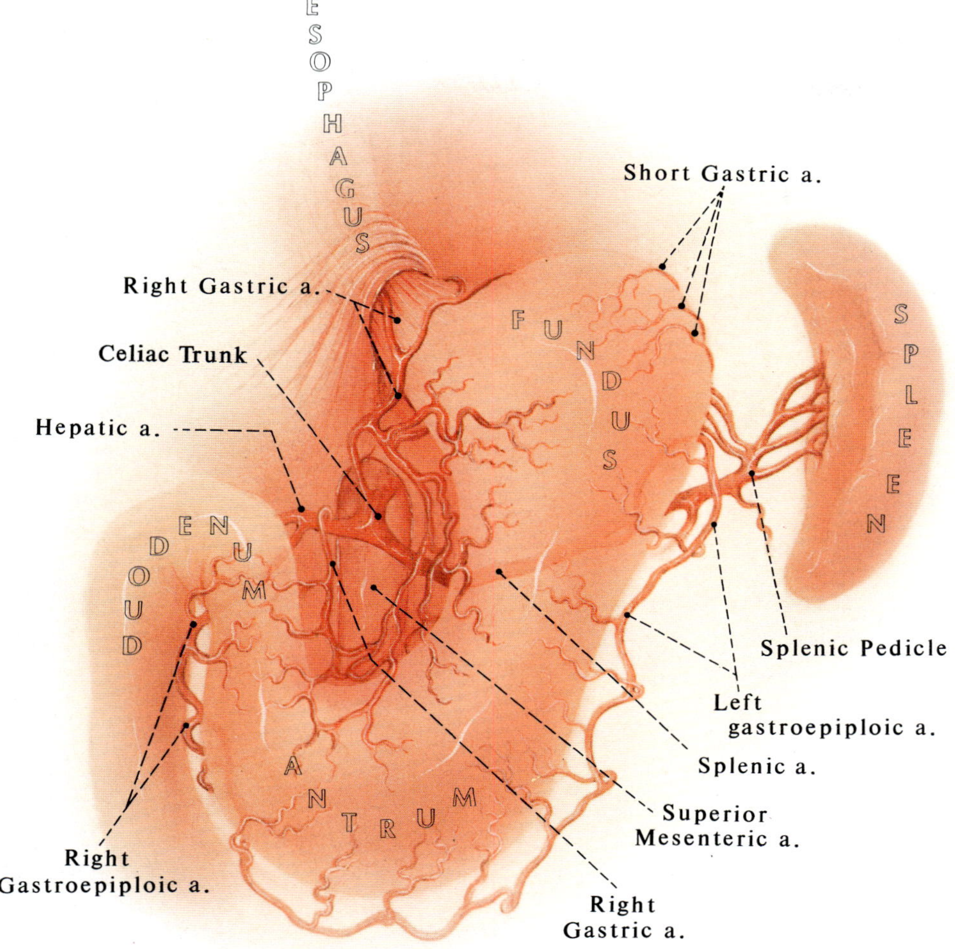

Arterial supply to the Stomach and Spleen

Physiology

The physiology of the stomach has intrigued investigators for many centuries and remains highly intricate. From a surgical standpoint, the important physiologic aspects are (1) secretion, (2) motility, and, to a lesser extent, (3) digestion.

Secretion

The gastric mucosa, per se, is divided into three definite areas: (1) the cardiac area, the zone immediately surrounding the esophagogastric junction, contains cardiac glands that predominantly secrete mucus; (2) the fundocorporeal area, which encompasses most of the body and fundus, has glands composed of mucous cells, chief (zygomatic) cells, and parietal (oxyntic) cells that secrete mucus, pepsinogen, and hydrochloric acid and intrinsic factor, respectively; and (3) the antrum, the glands of which are similar to the mucus-producing glands in the fundic area but, in addition, contain small cells (G cells) that produce gastrin and chief cells that produce pepsinogen.

Figure 2-2

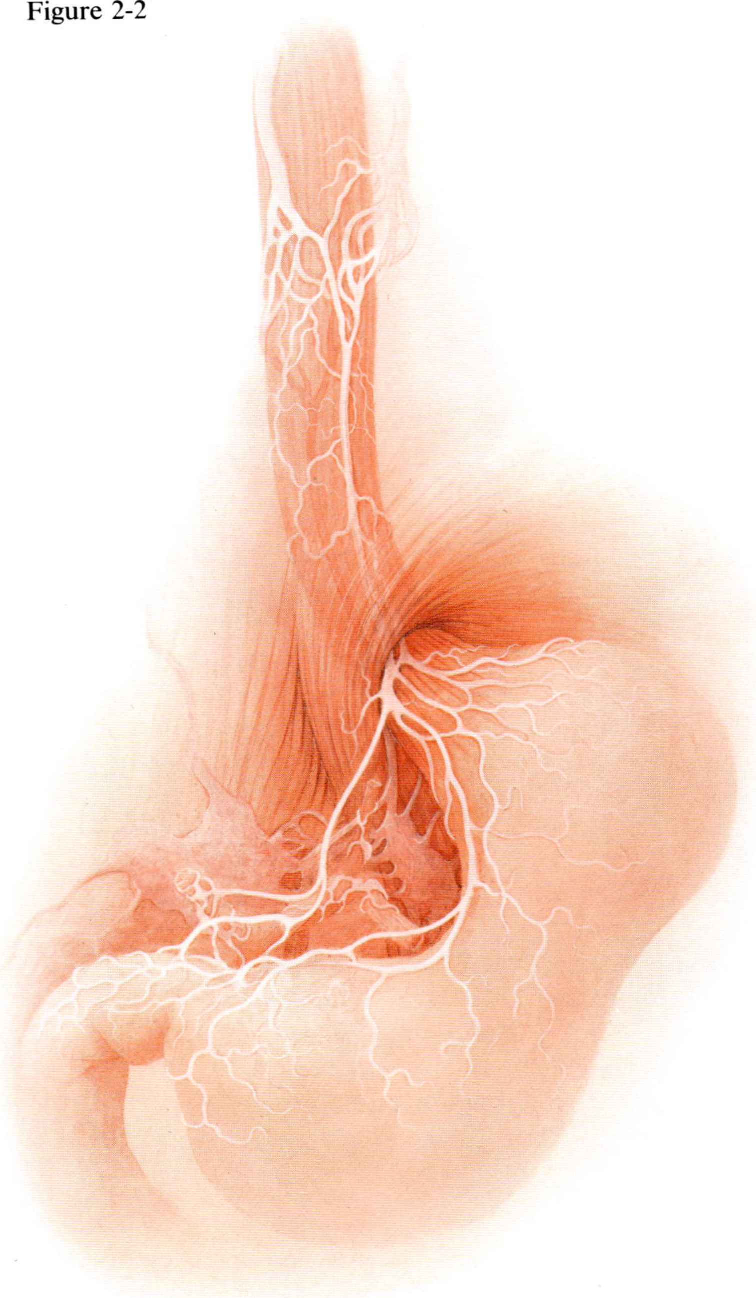

The normal daily secretion by the gastric mucosa varies between 500 and 2,000 ml. The regulation of gastric acid secretion involve two mechanisms: stimulation and inhibition.

The stimulation of gastric acid secretion is conveniently thought of as occurring by means of three separate phases (cephalic, gastric, and intestinal) in various combinations. In the cephalic phase, activation of the vagus nerves by the sight, smell, or thought of food stimulates the parietal cells, the chief cells, and the antral cells to secrete hydrochloric acid, pepsinogen, and gastrin, respectively. This phase is responsible for approximately 10% of gastric acid secretion. In the gastric phase, a small amount of gastric acid secretion is produced by the entry of food into the duodenum and upper jejunum. The exact mechanism of this phase is unknown, but it is probably due to the release of a gastrinlike substance that, in turn, stimulates the parietal cell mass.

The inhibition of gastric acid secretion involves two phases. In the vagal-antral phase, the removal of cerebral visual or olfactory stimulation of the vagus nerve decreases the stimulus. More important, however, is lowering of the antral pH, which inhibits the release of gastrin. In the intestinal phase, distention of the small bowel by the arrival of food sets into motion an inhibitory reflex via the sympathetic and parasympathetic nerves. In addition, inhibitory humoral factors—gastric inhibitory polypeptide and the prostaglandins—are released.

Motility

For the consideration of motility, the stomach can conveniently be thought of as being composed of proximal and distal halves. The proximal half acts as a reservoir and controls the emptying of liquids from the stomach by sustained tonic contraction, while the distal half acts as both a grinder and a separator and basically controls the emptying of solids.

A gastric pacemaker has been localized to the midbody of the stomach along the greater curvature. Pacesetter potentials are generated by this pacemaker at a frequency of about 3 cycles/min. These potentials travel both circumferentially and distally and increase in both amplitude and velocity as they approach the pylorus. These electrical waves trigger peristaltic contractions in the distal corpus and antrum that mix and grind digestible solids until they are particles of only a few millimeters in size. The pyloric sphincter opens to allow liquids and small solids to pass. As soon as the bolus has passed, it closes to prevent duodenal reflux, and it then reopens. Each peristaltic wave empties 3 to 6 ml of chyme into the duodenum. Gastric emptying is mainly a forward thrust; little "to-and-fro" movement occurs across the pylorus.

The stomach has a remarkable capacity for dilatation. With distention, the gastric wall relaxes to allow for a great increase in intragastric volume with little alteration in intragastric pressure. The ease and rapidity of gastric emptying are directly related to the liquidity of gastric chyme. Duodenal receptors, by neurohormonal mechanisms, decrease gastric emptying by decreasing gastric motility. In addition, gastric emptying is influenced by many other factors, including sectioning of the vagal trunks, duodenal distention, osmolality and acidity of the duodenal chyme, quantity of protein and fat in the chyme, and the competence or incompetence of the pyloric sphincter.

3 Duodenal Ulcers

Jon A. van Heerden

Etiology

When the delicate balance between the acid-pepsin secretion of the stomach and the mucosal resistance of the duodenum goes awry, acid-peptic autodigestion of the duodenal mucosa (duodenal ulceration) ensues. The cause of this lesion is highly complex and multifactorial (Fig. 3-1 and 3-2). Stimulatory factors include increased acid secretion (even though most patients with duodenal ulcer have gastric acid levels within the normal range), rapid gastric emptying, increased secretion of pepsin, inappropriate gastrin release, decreased inhibition of acid secretion and gastrin release, and inadequate feedback inhibition of gastric acid secretion by possible deficiencies in vasoactive intestinal polypeptide, somatostatin, and glucagon. Mucosal resistance (cytoprotection) is equally complex and is less well understood. Mucosal resistance seems to be prostaglandin related—prostaglandin E_2 in particular—and may involve increased mucosal blood supply, protection of the mucosal barrier, and stimulation of cyclic adenosine monophosphate formation.

Better understood are the precise pathologic conditions that lead to duodenal ulceration. These conditions include islet cell tumors (gastrinomas) and antral G-cell hyperplasia; both lesions mediate ulcer formation by means of excessive release of gastrin. In addition, duodenal ulceration seems to be associated with a genetic predisposition, as evidenced by the preponderance of patients with duodenal ulceration who have blood group O and the well-known association of the autosomally dominant multiple endocrine neoplasia type I syndrome and the hyperpepsinogenemia I syndrome.

Treatment

In patients with duodenal ulceration, the classic indications for surgical intervention (which is required in approximately 10% to 15% of patients) are (1) gastric outlet obstruction (Fig. 3-3), (2) duodenal perforation (Fig. 3-4), (3) duodenal hemorrhage (Fig. 3-5), (4) posterior pancreatic penetration (Fig. 3-6), and (5) intractability.

During the past 10 to 15 years, the incidence of duodenal ulceration has steadily, but unexplainably, decreased. The H_2 antagonists have been in-

Figure 3-1

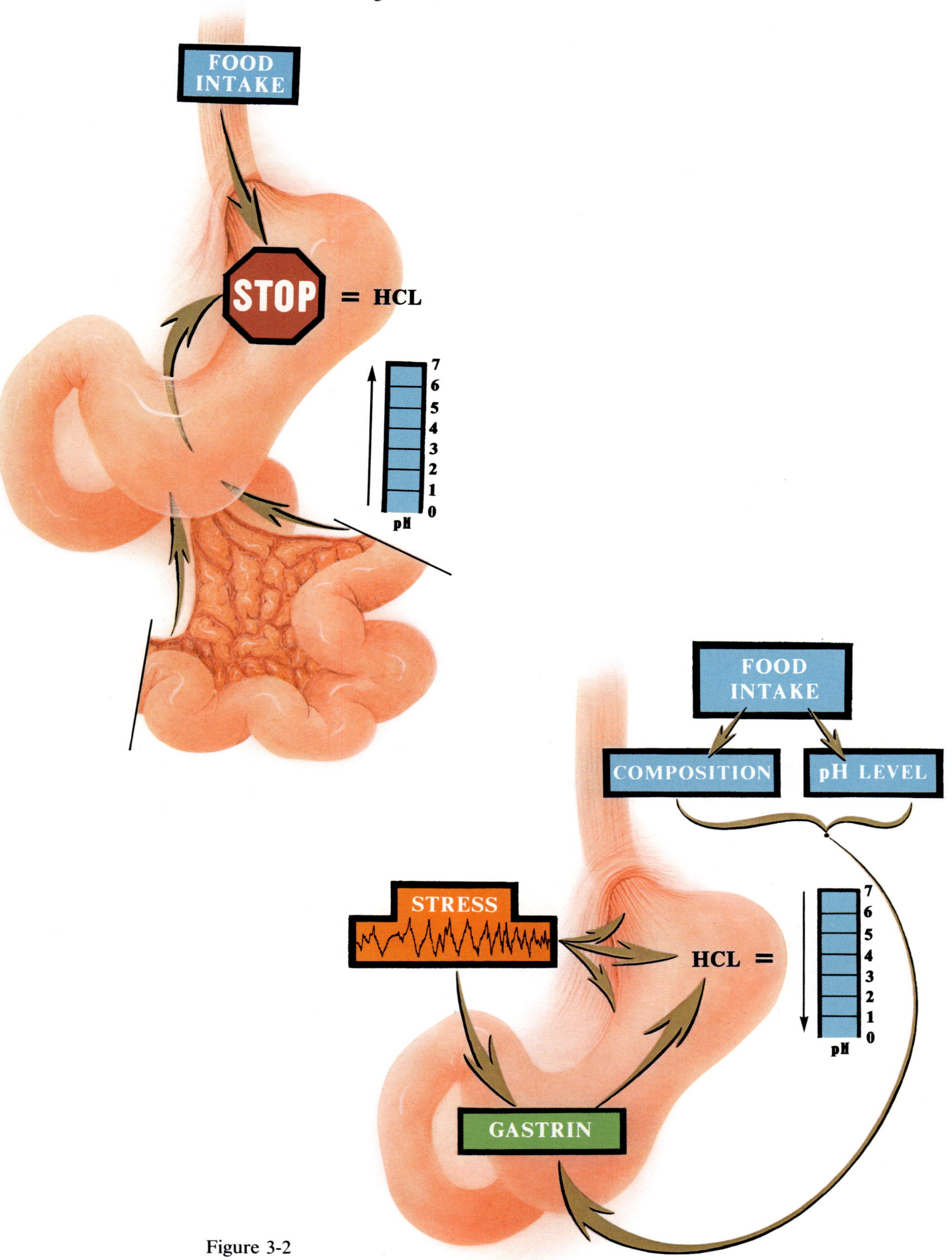

Figure 3-2

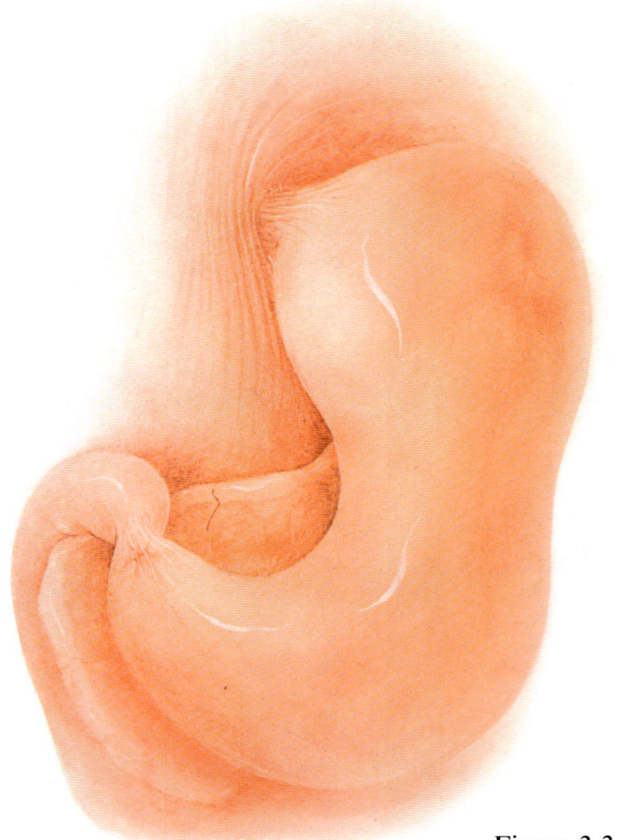

Figure 3-3

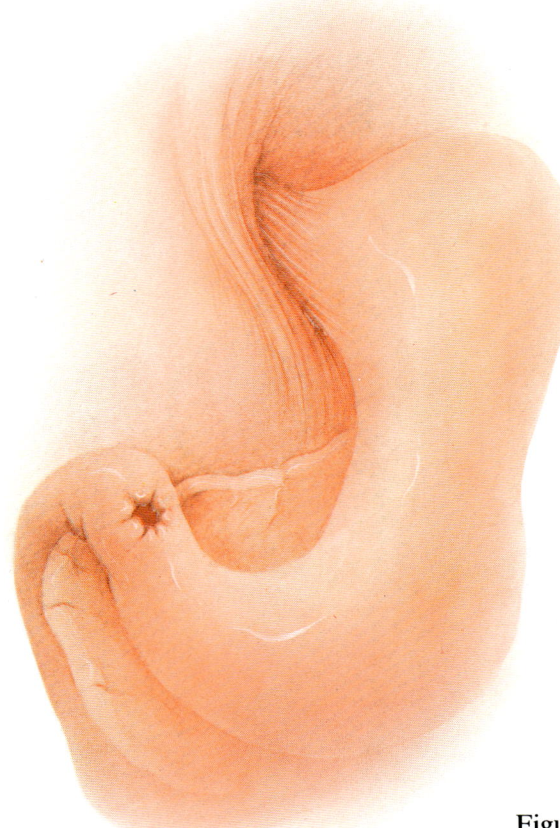

Figure 3-4

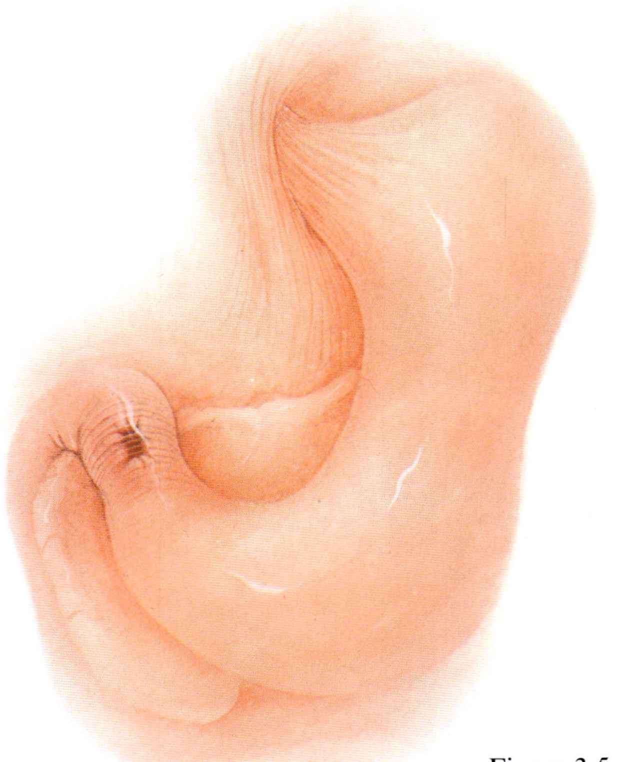

Figure 3-5

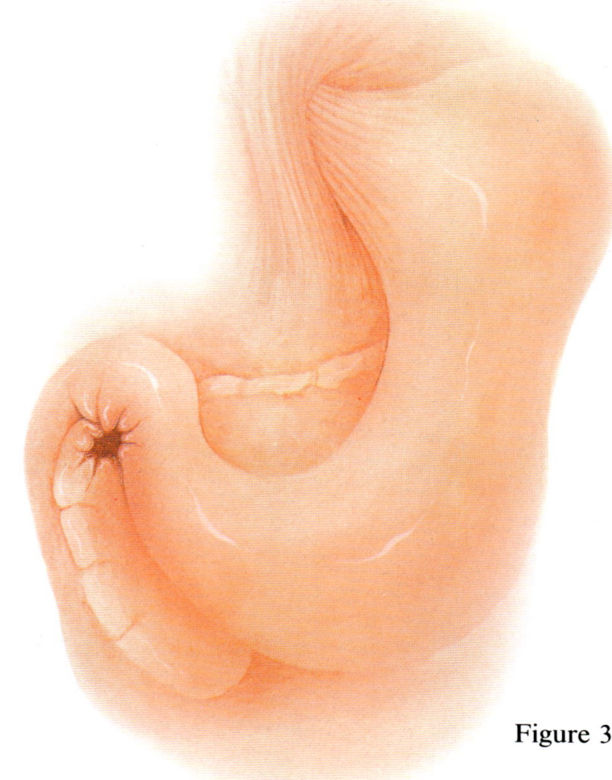

Figure 3-6

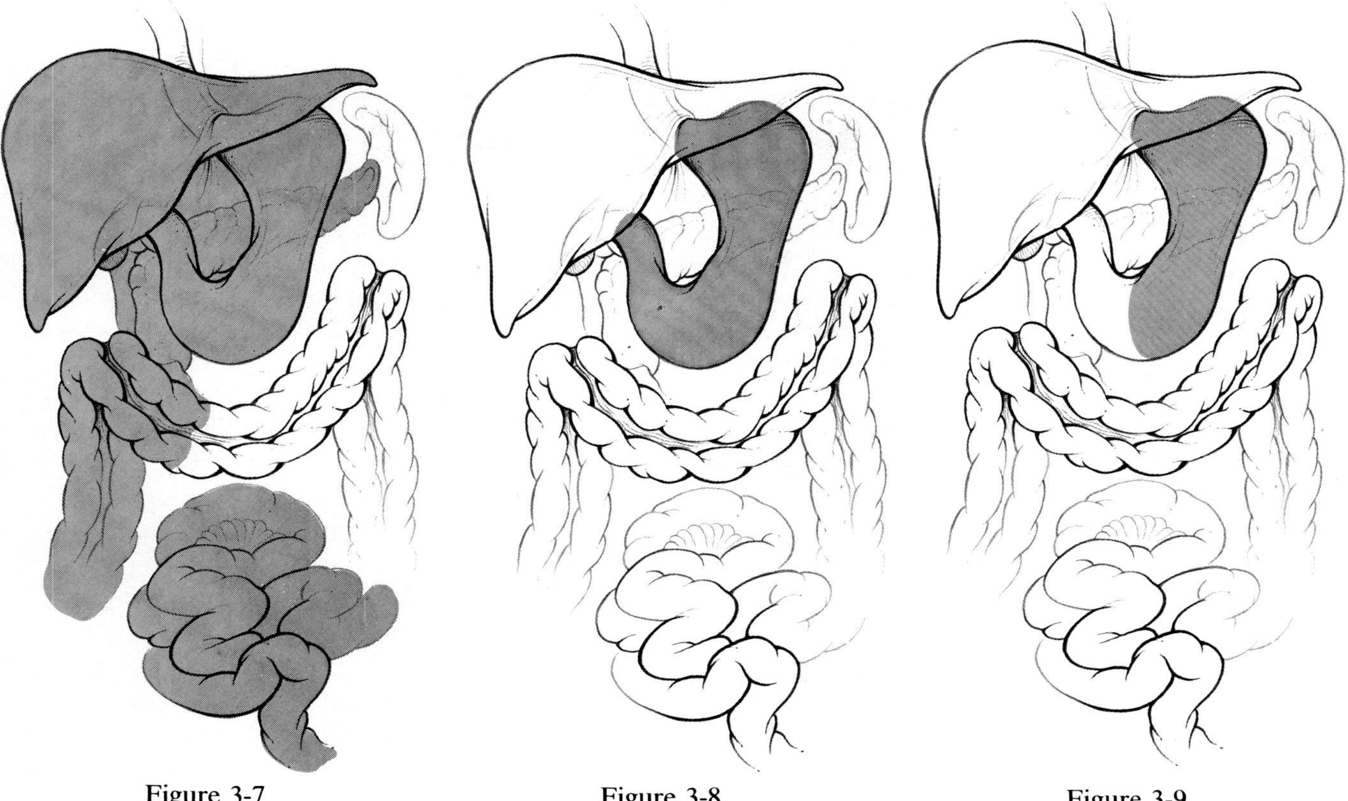

Figure 3-7 Figure 3-8 Figure 3-9

criminated in this reduction; this charge is somewhat erroneous, however, because these antagonists seem to have had no influence on the actual incidence of the disease. Passaro has suggested that if the current rate of decline were to continue, no operations for duodenal ulceration would be performed by the year 1992!

Types

Sir Hennig Ogilvie aptly stated, "Every operation for duodenal ulceration is a success until it is found out." This prophetic statement is exemplified by the continuing changes in the refinement of the treatment of this puzzling entity that have occurred during this century. Surgical treatment has ranged from simple gastroenterostomy (popularized by the Mayo brothers and used in the 1920s and 1930s) to subtotal gastric resection (used in the 1940s and 1950s) to proximal gastric vagotomy (popularized by Holle and Goligher and used in the 1970s and 1980s).

Despite this continuing evolution, physicians currently uniformly agree, mainly due to the early pioneering work of the late Dr. Lester Dragstedt, that some type of vagotomy should be an integral part of the treatment of duodenal ulceration. The type of vagotomy may be (1) truncal (complete) (Fig. 3-7), with resultant denervation of the stomach, duodenum, entire small intestine, right half of the colon, liver, gallbladder, and pancreas; (2) total gastric (selective) (Fig. 3-8), with denervation of the stomach only; or (3) proximal gastric (highly selective) (Fig. 3-9), with denervation of the parietal cell mass only.

Surgeons have been instrumental in the refinement of vagotomy techniques, trying continuously to achieve a good balance among a low operative mortality; minimal immediate postoperative morbidity; a low recurrence rate; and acceptable long-term morbidity—diarrhea and the dumping syndrome in particular.

On the basis of a survey of the literature up to 1984, the following conclusions might be made regarding the various operations that are available for the treatment of duodenal ulceration: (1) the operation with the highest postoperative mortality in a good-risk patient is gastric resection; (2) the operation with the highest recurrence rate is truncal vagotomy and pyloroplasty; (3) the operation with the lowest incidence of postoperative diarrhea and dumping is proximal gastric vagotomy; (4) the operation with the lowest postoperative mortality is proximal gastric vagotomy; and (5) the operation with the lowest incidence of recurrence is truncal vagotomy and antrectomy.

Proximal Gastric (Highly Selective) Vagotomy. Exposure for this operation is best obtained through either an upper midline (Fig. 3-10) or a transverse epigastric incision (Fig. 3-11) in which extension to the right is favored. Of great value for exposure when either of these incisions is used is the so-called upper-hand or third-arm mechanical retractor, which increases the anteroposterior diameter of the epigastrium (Fig. 3-12). The use of this retractor, in addition to a Balfour retractor when a midline incision is used (Fig. 3-13), affords excellent exposure. Elevation of the head of the operating table 15° to 20° is advisable. The technical ease of this operation is largely dependent on body size, the amount of fat in the gastrohepatic omentum, and the anteroposterior diameter of the epigastrium. In most patients, careful scrutiny of the gastrohepatic omentum in the supra-antral position will clearly reveal the "crow's foot," which is the termination of the nerves of Latarjet (see Fig. 2-2). If excessive fat is present in this omentum, however, this termination may not be visible. Alternatively, the hepatic branch of the anterior vagus nerve is almost always visible to the right of the esophagogastric junction and acts as an excellent landmark in the obese patient (see Fig. 2-2).

An initial step in the performance of a proximal gastric vagotomy is identification of both the anterior and the posterior vagal trunks above the esophagogastric junction and placement of silk sutures around these trunks. This step was popularized by Goligher, but it is probably dispensable once sufficient experience is gained. The surgeon's left hand is the dominant hand in this operation and should be placed into the lesser sac via the avascular portion of the gastrohepatic omentum, which is to the right of the nerves of Latarjet (Fig. 3-14). With traction applied by this hand, which should remain in this position throughout the operation, in opposition to traction applied on the stomach with a Babcock clamp or clamps by an assistant, tension is created on the gastrohepatic omentum, and visualization of the nerves and vessels to be sectioned is excellent.

Dissection should commence with division of the "heel" of the "crow's foot," usually 6 to 7 cm proximal to the pylorus on the lesser curvature (Fig. 3-15). Dissection then proceeds proximally by serially ligating and dividing both the anterior and posterior leaves of the gastrohepatic omentum close to the stomach. This rather tedious and repetitive process may be speeded by using silver hemoclips, but they have been proved to be inefficient because they are often dislodged during higher dissection and thus cause unnecessary and rather troublesome hematoma formation. As dissection proceeds superiorly, the hepatic branch of the anterior vagus nerve is kept clearly in view. Dissection proceeds tangentially across the esophagogastric junction toward the angle of His. Once this angle is

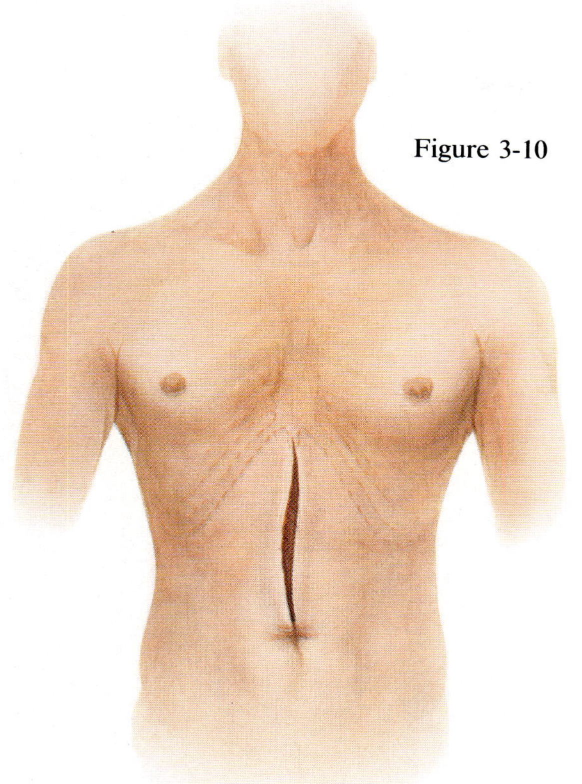
Figure 3-10

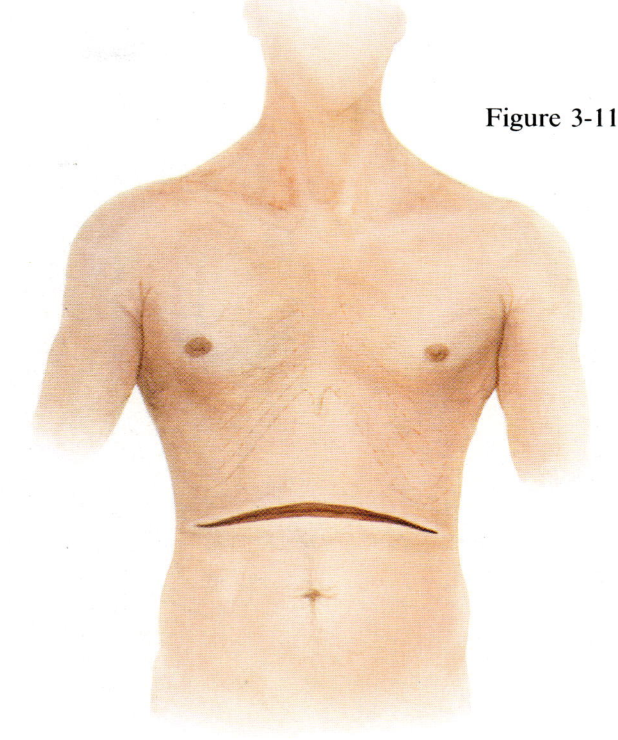
Figure 3-11

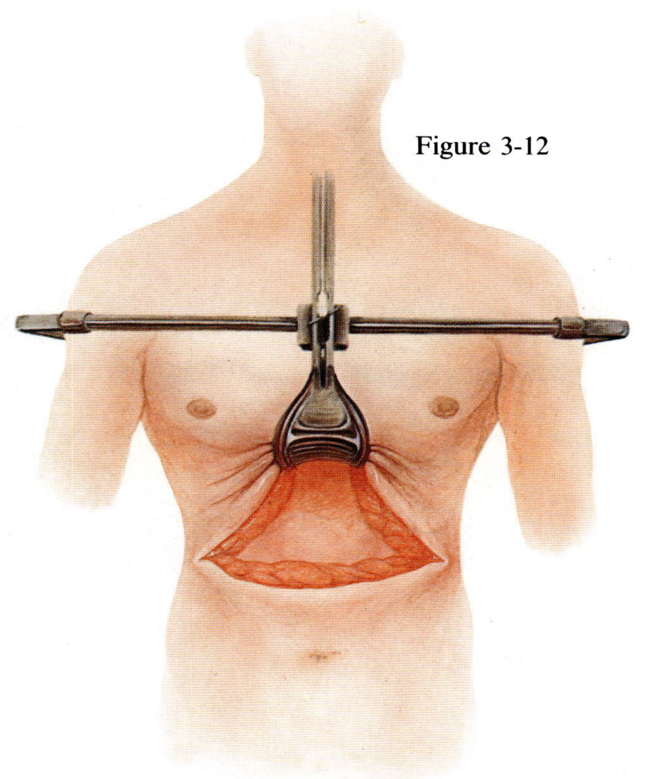
Figure 3-12

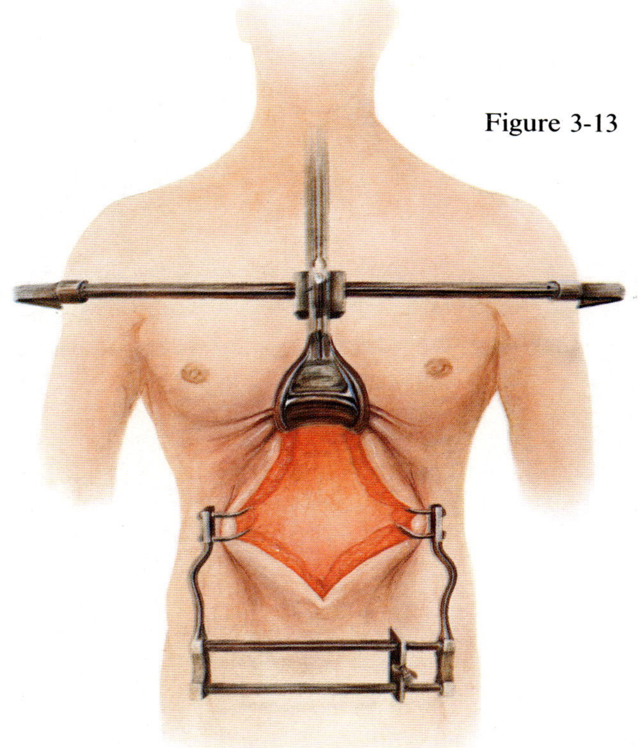
Figure 3-13

Figure 3-14

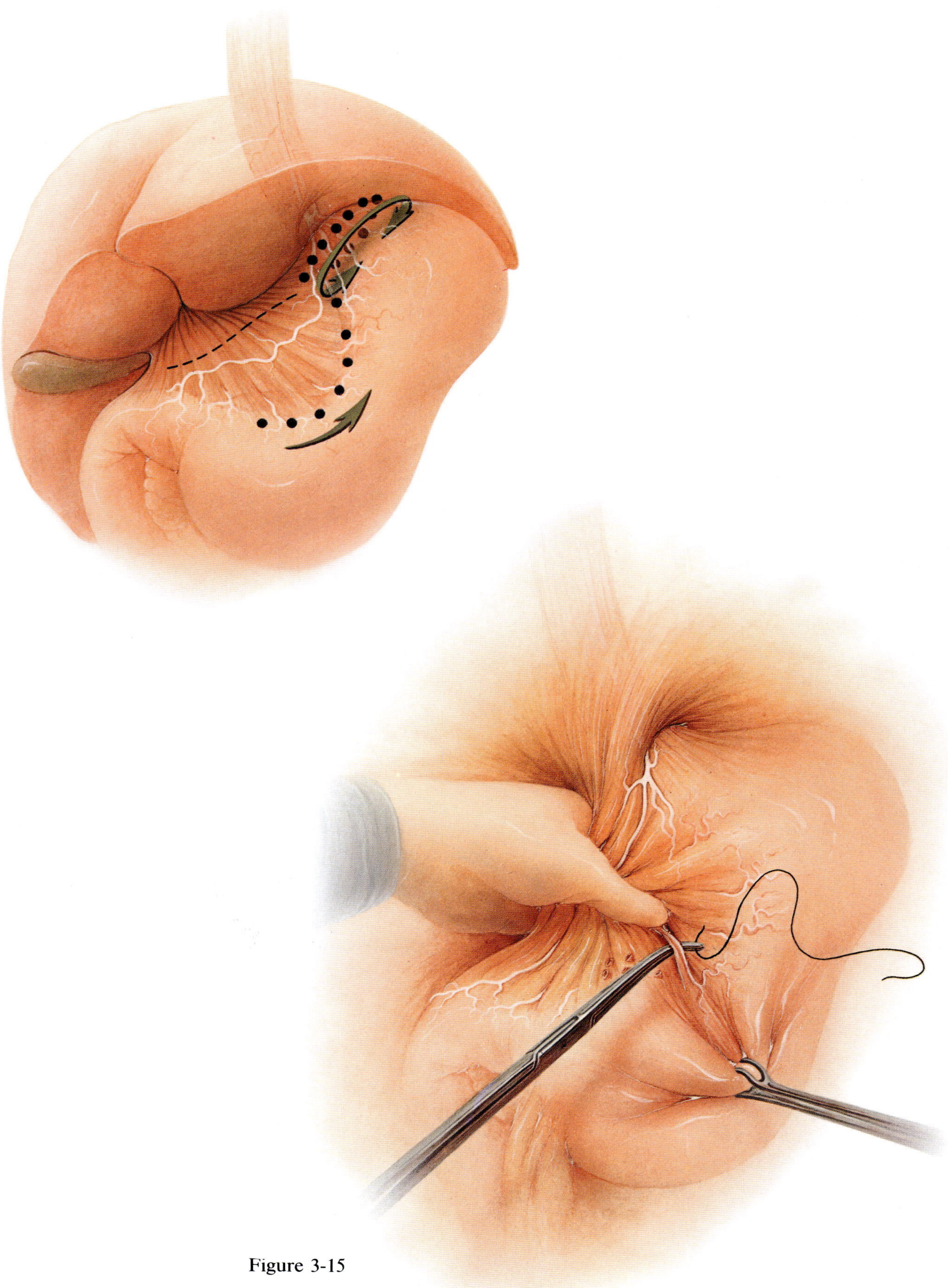

Figure 3-15

Figure 3-16

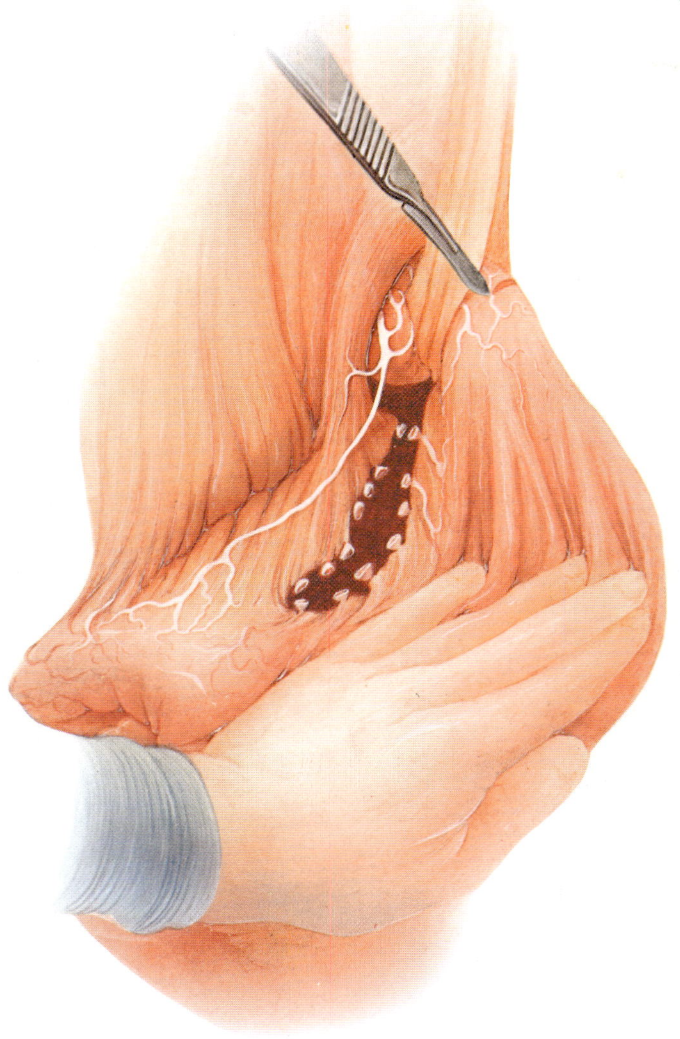

reached, the esophagus needs to be "denuded" for a distance of at least 6 cm (Fig. 3-16). This is accomplished by carefully dividing the small vagal fibers circumferentially with the scalpel or by electrocautery to thus allow a proximal "sweep" to occur.

By encircling the lower esophagus with either a Penrose drain or umbilical tape, anterior traction allows visualization of the posterior aspect of the esophagogastric junction and fundus of the stomach. This maneuver is of importance in seeking a rare, but important, posterior vagal branch to the fundus, which has been termed the criminal nerve of Grassi. Complete proximal gastric vagotomy is ensured if the first one or two short gastric vessels are divided and, in addition, the greater omentum is divided halfway along the greater curvature to interrupt the gastroepiploic vessels. This step ensures division of the so-called nerve of Rosati, which, at times, might be responsible for incomplete parietal cell denervation. The lesser curvature may be reperitonealized with interrupted silk sutures. Theoretically, this measure not only prevents any subsequent reestablishment of vagal innervation to this area but also may invert small areas of necrosis of the lesser curvature that are most likely due to inadvertent inclusion of part of the wall of the lesser curvature in surgical ties. This technical

Figure 3-17

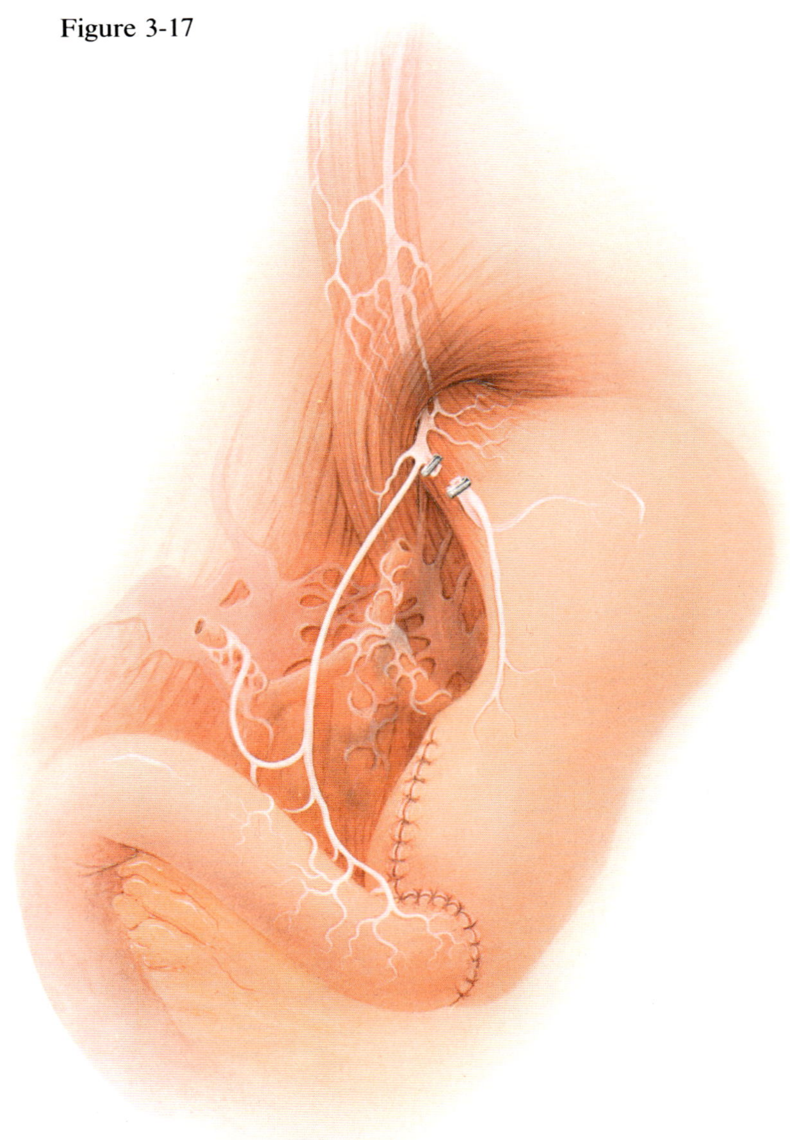

error is probably the cause for the rarely reported instance of necrosis of the lesser curvature after proximal gastric vagotomy.

The principal tests for the intraoperative monitoring of vagal completeness during proximal gastric vagotomy are the Grassi and the Burge (mucosal pH mapping) tests. Although little data can be found to substantiate the value of the Grassi test, the same cannot be said of the Burge test. Data suggest that the recurrence of ulcer in patients with positive results of the Burge test is almost 5 times that in patients with negative results. No form of gastric drainage is needed after this procedure, despite its advocacy by Holle. The addition of either pyloroplasty or gastroenterostomy to proximal gastric vagotomy negates the beneficial effects of this operation as they relate to both diarrhea and dumping. In patients with an element of obstruction of the pyloric channel, dilation with a large-bore gastric tube or Hegar dilators has proved adequate in selected instances.

Total Gastric (Selective) Vagotomy. As the name implies, all of the vagal fibers to the stomach, distal to the hepatic and celiac branches, are divided (Fig. 3-17). This operation requires an emptying procedure—either a pylo-

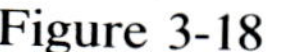
Figure 3-18

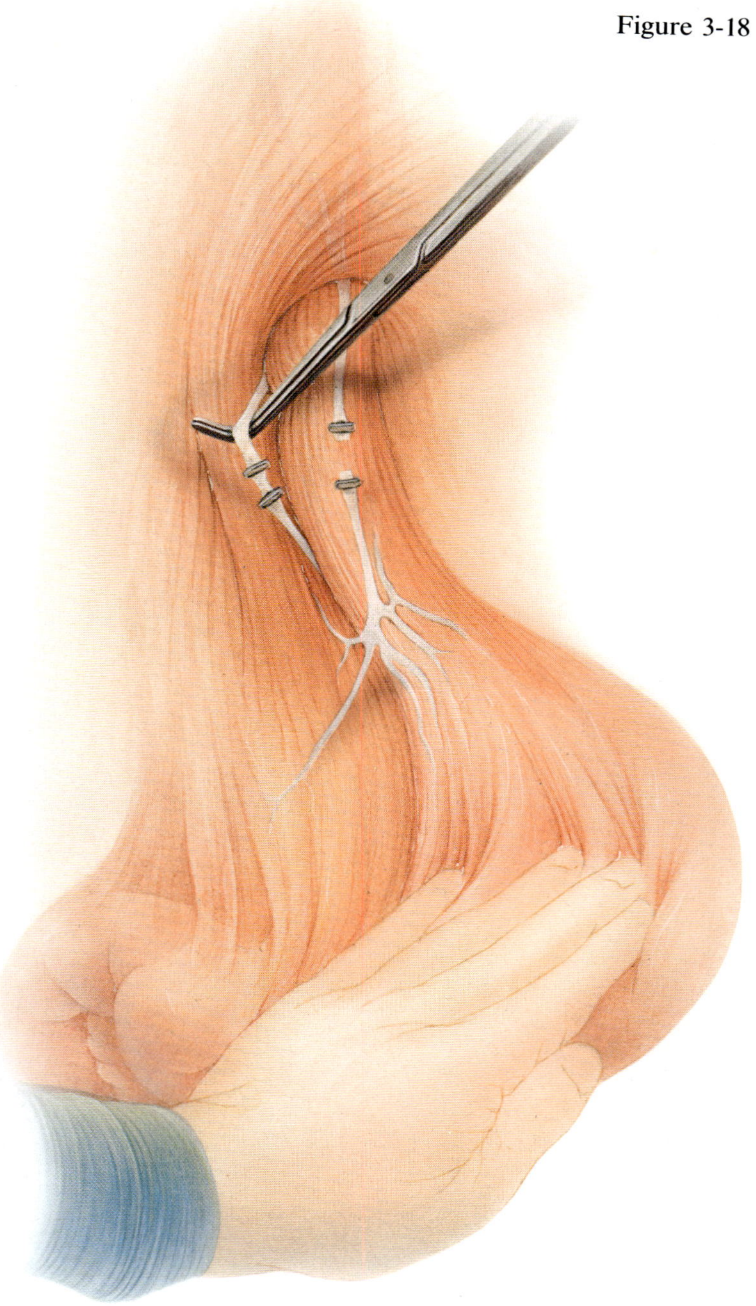

roplasty or antrectomy. Because of this requirement, this operation has little, if any, advantage over a truncal vagotomy. This procedure has not gained wide popularity.

Truncal (Complete) Vagotomy. Either an upper midline or a transverse epigastric incision with liberal use of the third-arm retractor is suitable. The key to truncal vagotomy is exposure. Exposure is best obtained by superior and *anterior* retraction of the left lobe of the liver and anterior abdominal wall with a deep retractor, such as a Harrington retractor, and inferior retraction on the body of the stomach by the surgeon's left hand placed on a folded sponge (Fig. 3-18). The placement of this hand is the key to the operation. Although the anterior vagal trunk is intimately related to the anterior surface of the esophagus, in which it may be imbedded

Figure 3-19

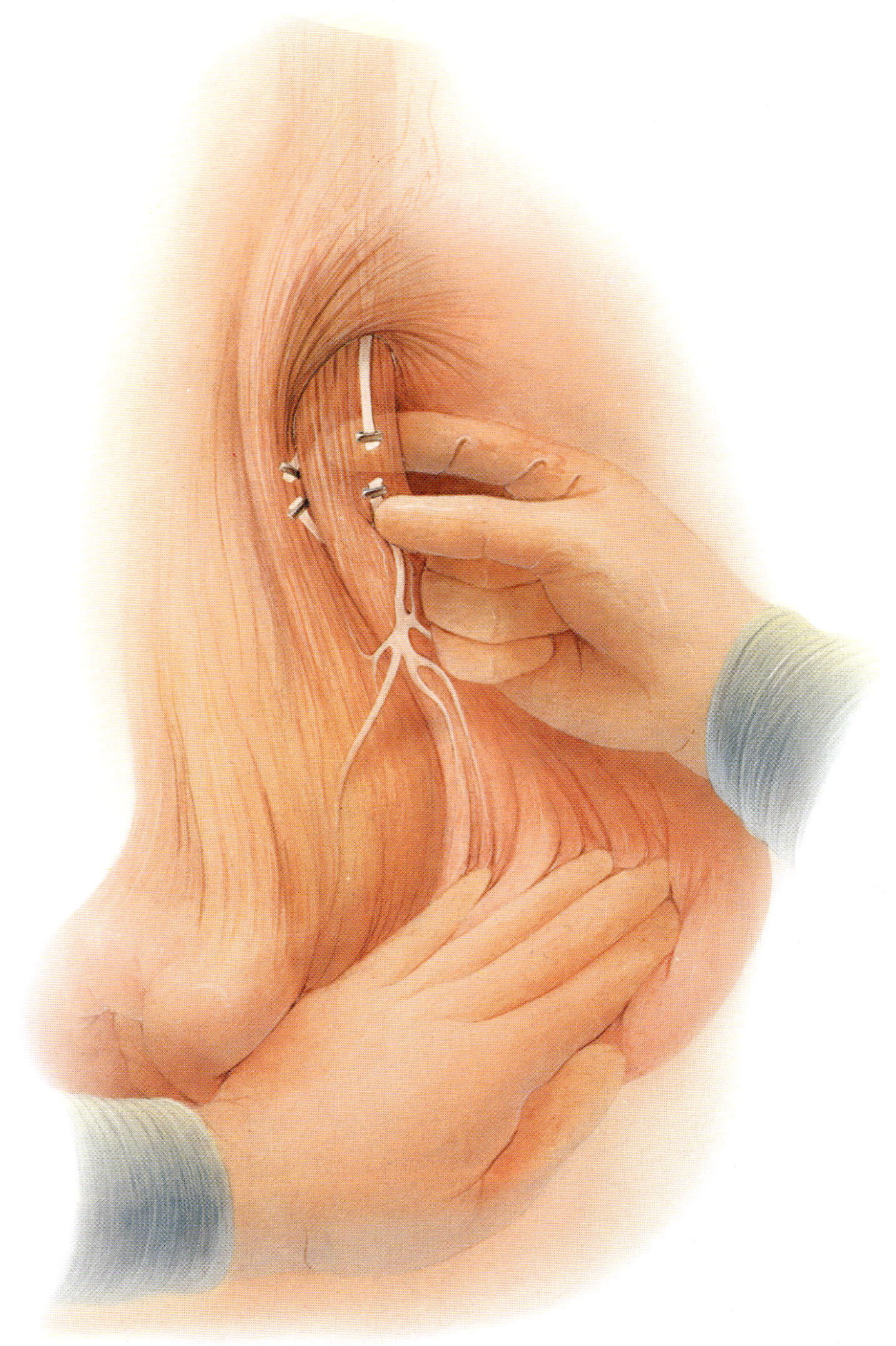

(2 o'clock position), the posterior vagal trunk (7 o'clock position) is clearly separated from the esophagus by a distance of 1 cm to 1.5 cm. The method of division, by clipping or ligation (Fig. 3-19), is perhaps immaterial, but histologic examination is not. One of the most frequent causes for an incomplete truncal vagotomy is the absence of frozen-section identification of nerve trunks. The surgeon should not be satisfied after the two major trunks are divided because multiple other small and not insignificant branches are often encountered if carefully sought, especially on the anterior aspect of the esophagus.

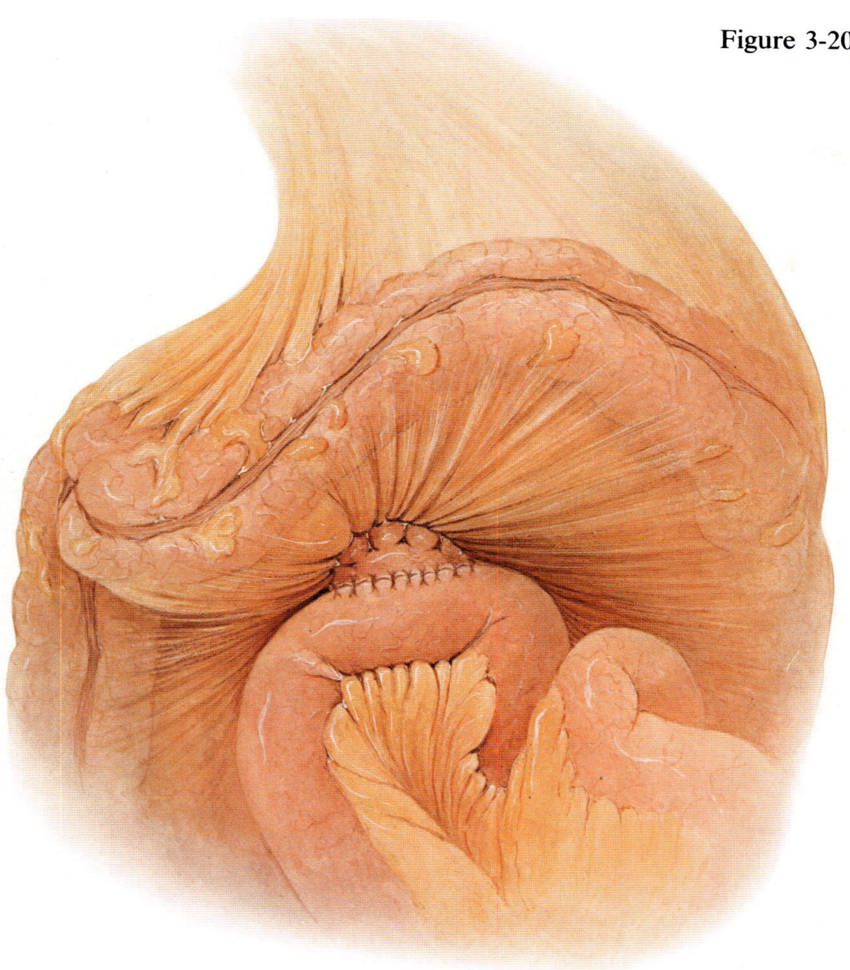

Figure 3-20

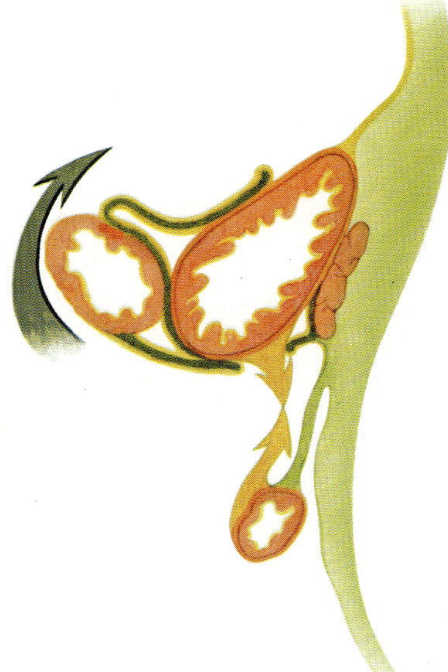

Figure 3-21

Gastrojejunostomy. This anastomosis can be performed in either the retrocolic (Fig. 3-20 and 3-21) or antecolic (Fig. 3-22 and 3-23) position. The advantage of the retrocolic position is the very short afferent limb, which may be advantageous in operations for peptic ulceration. The avascular spot in the transverse mesocolon, just to the left of the middle colic vessels, is an ideal site for the placement of this anastomosis. In the retrocolic position, the gastric wall (Fig. 3-21), per se, and not the small bowel, should be sutured to the edges of the mesocolic defect to prevent possible retrogastric (Peterson's) herniation. Antecolic gastrojejunostomy is preferable for pancreatic malignant disease. Whether the anastomosis is constructed in an isoperistaltic or antiperistaltic position is immaterial from a functional standpoint, and this decision should be individualized.

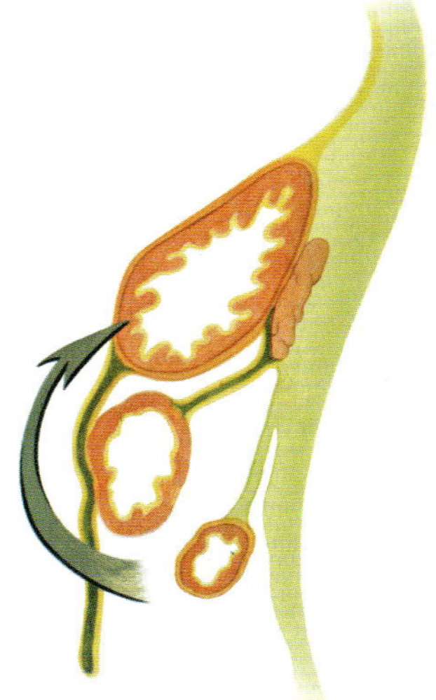

Figure 3-22

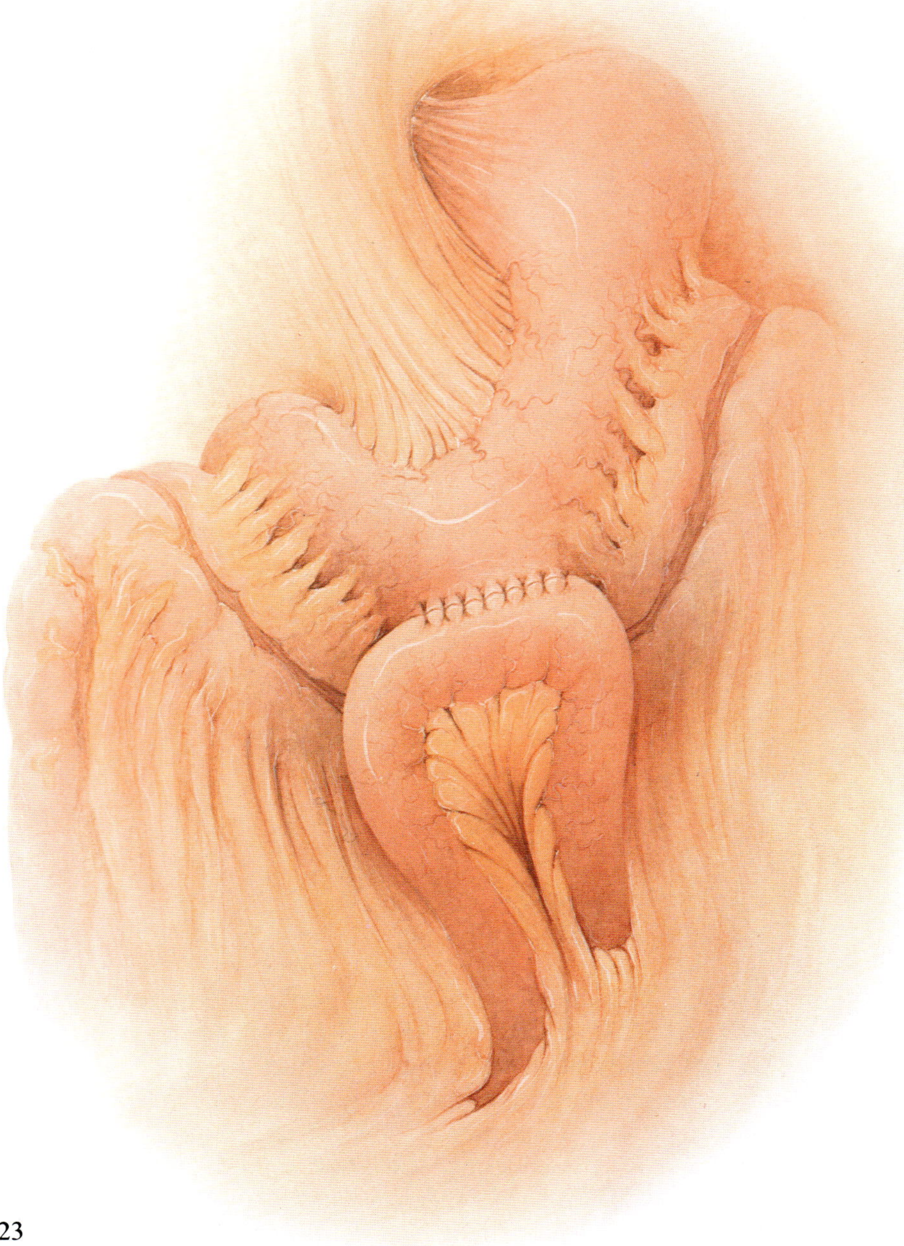

Figure 3-23

Pyloroplasty. Three classic pyloroplasties are used surgically to establish gastric outlet drainage: Heineke-Mikulicz (Fig. 3-24), Finney (Fig. 3-25 through 3-28), and Jaboulay (Fig. 3-29 and 3-30). The most frequently used is the Heineke-Mikulicz pyloroplasty with the Weinberg modification. The longitudinal gastroduodenal incision should be approximately 8 cm in length and should be roughly divided into 4.5 cm on the gastric aspect and 3.5 cm on the duodenal aspect (Fig. 3-31). This procedure entails closure with a single layer of interrupted nonabsorbable sutures. It is important to place these sutures approximately at a 60° angle. With this placement, entry into the serosa occurs 3 to 4 mm from the cut edge but only a millimeter (at most) of mucosa is included (Fig. 3-32).

Figure 3-24

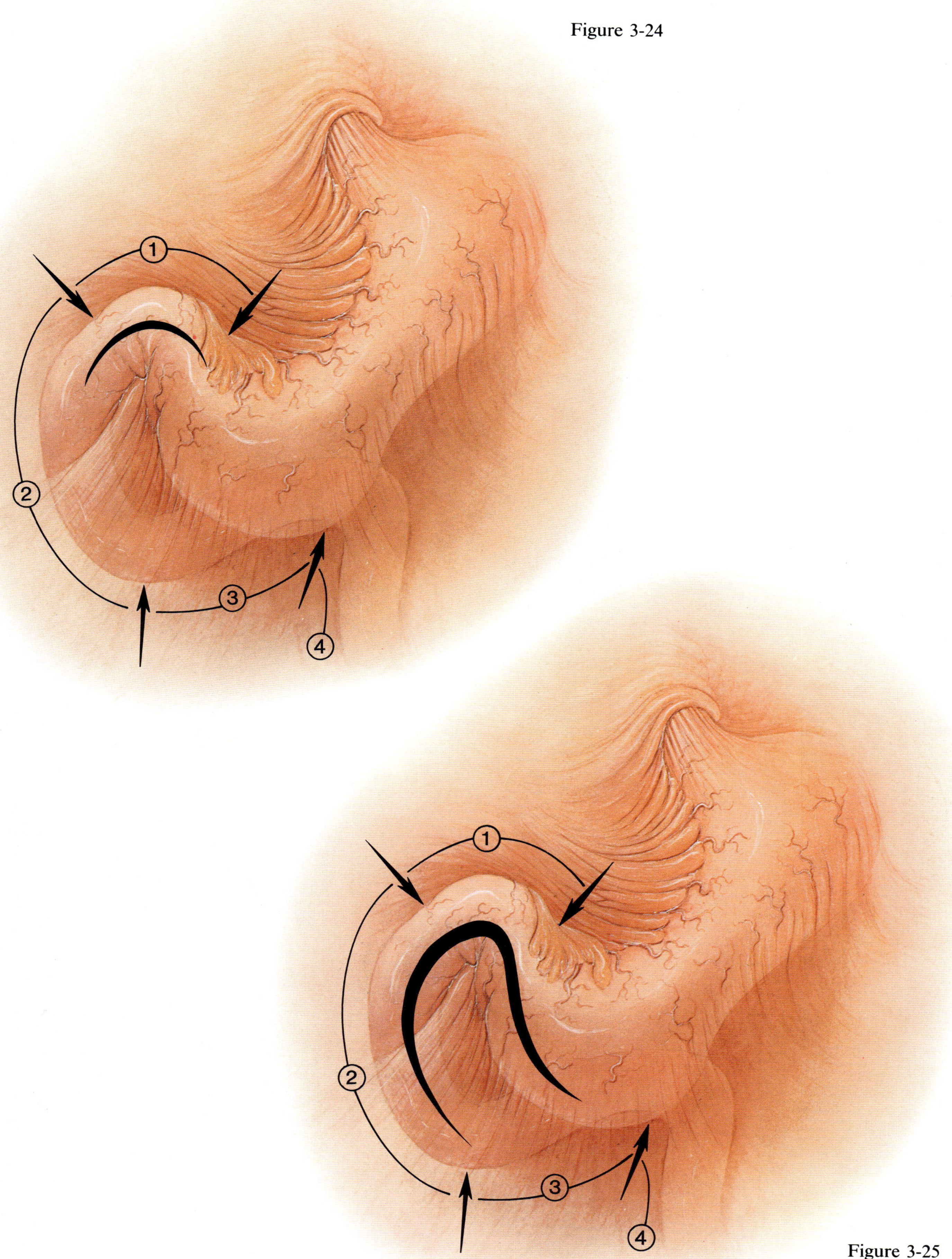

Figure 3-25

Figure 3-26

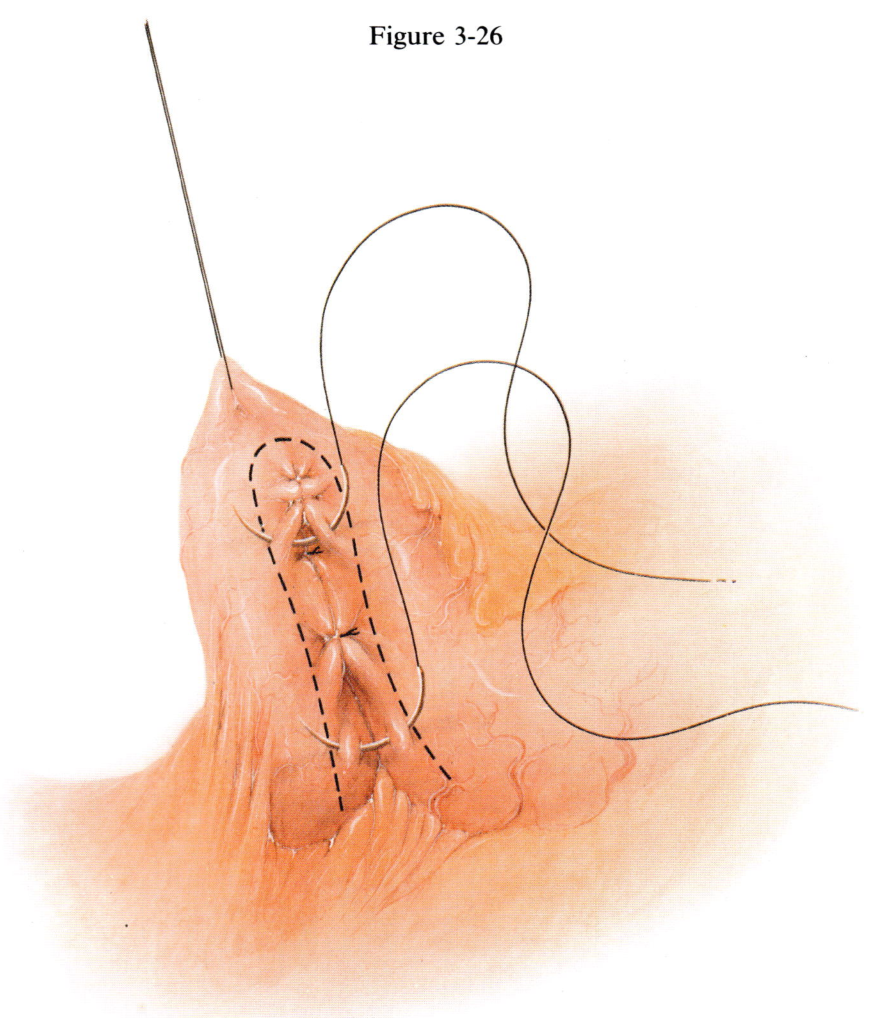

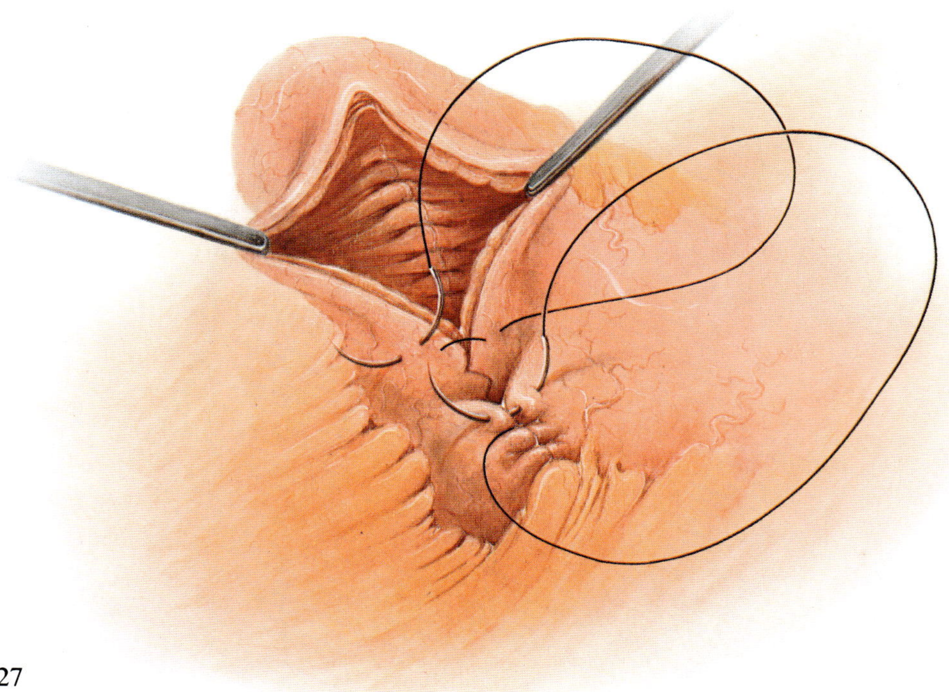

Figure 3-27

Figure 3-28

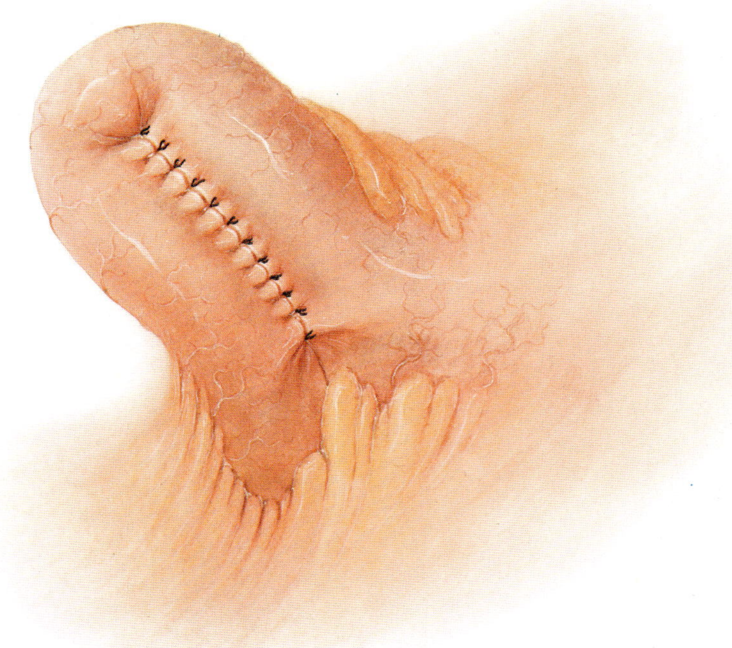

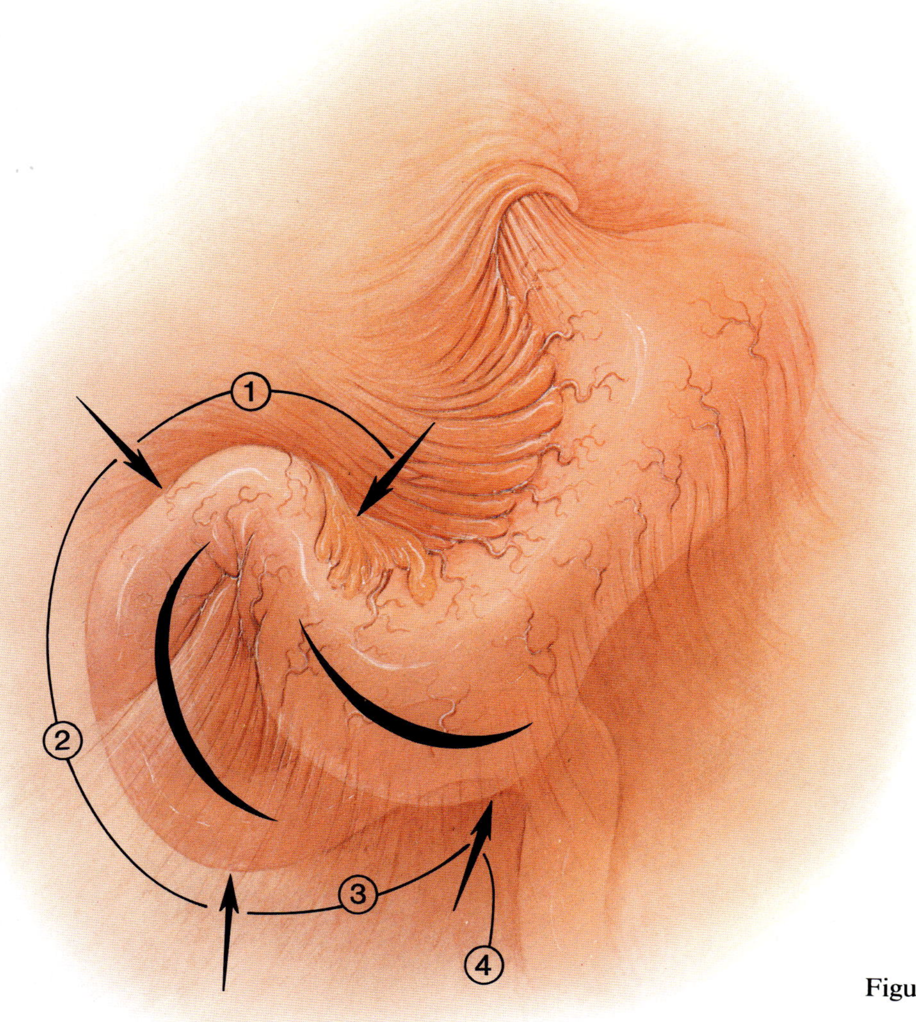

Figure 3-29

Figure 3-30

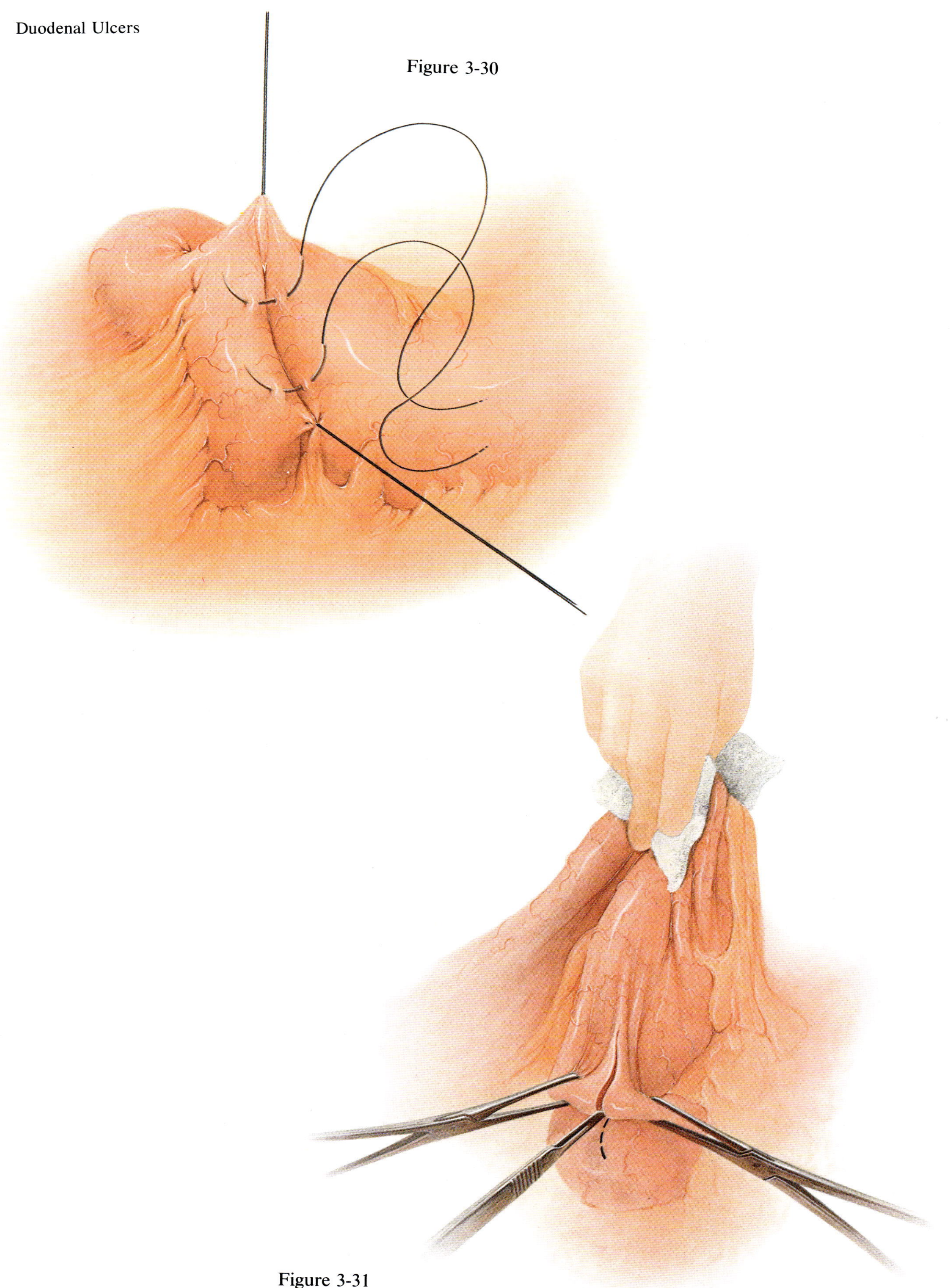

Figure 3-31

Figure 3-32

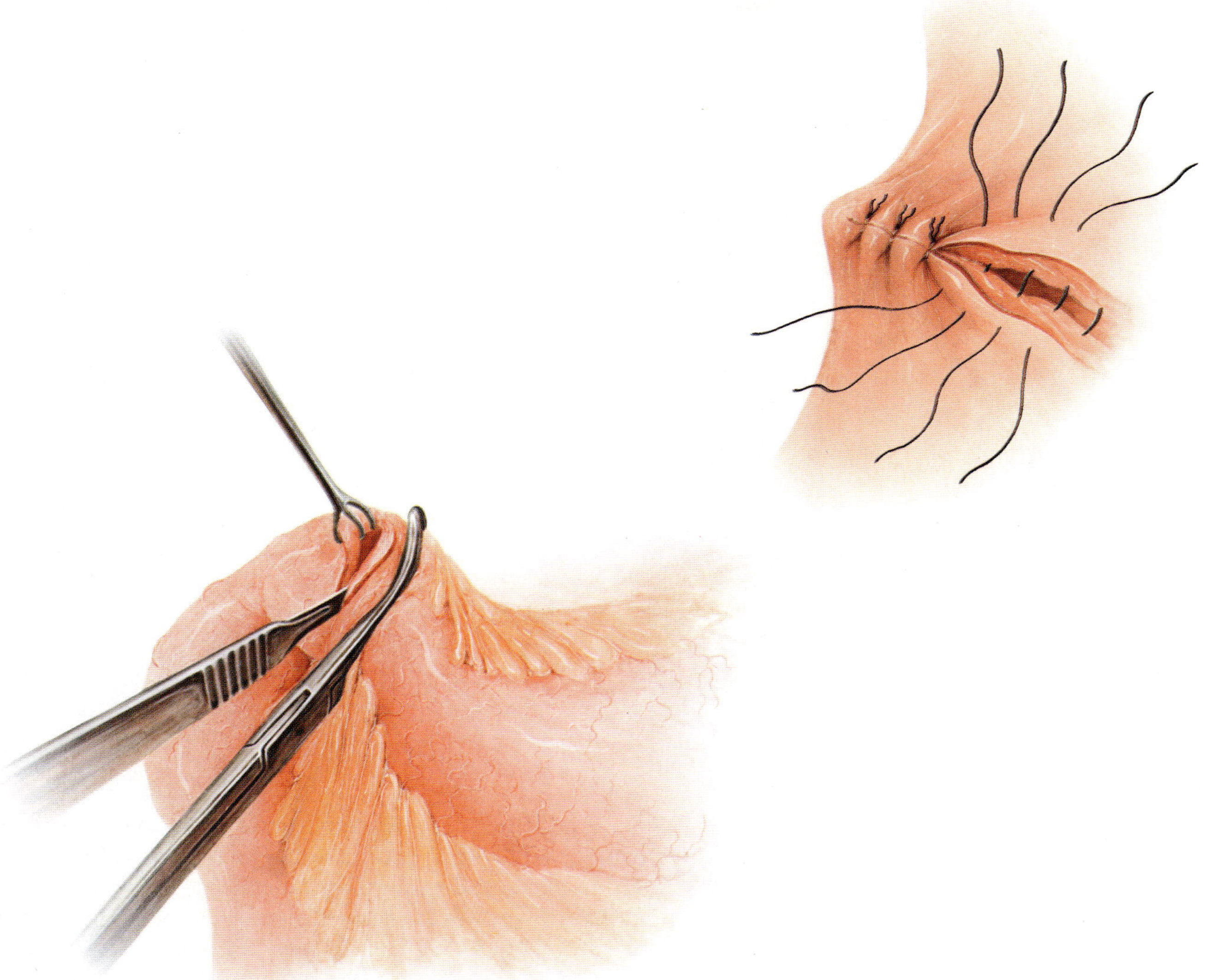

Figure 3-33

Antrectomy. The important technical points in the performance of an antrectomy are as follows.

The right gastric artery should be ligated by remaining close to the superior aspect of the first portion of the duodenum. By doing so, any potential injury to the common hepatic artery or common bile duct is unlikely.

When a great deal of fibrosis is present, histologic (frozen-section) identification of the duodenal mucosa is particularly important. Unless this examination is done, a retained gastric antrum, with its ulcerogenic potential, becomes a real possibility, particularly if a gastrojejunostomy is performed in the reconstruction.

No clamps should be placed across the duodenum. Instead, the duodenum may be stabilized with either Babcock or Allis clamps (Fig. 3-33). Partial closure of the divided stomach (Schoemaker [Billroth I] or Hofmeister [Billroth II] modification) is greatly facilitated by using a Payr clamp (Fig. 3-34). This closure should be secure and is best performed with two rows of running absorbable sutures reinforced by an outer layer

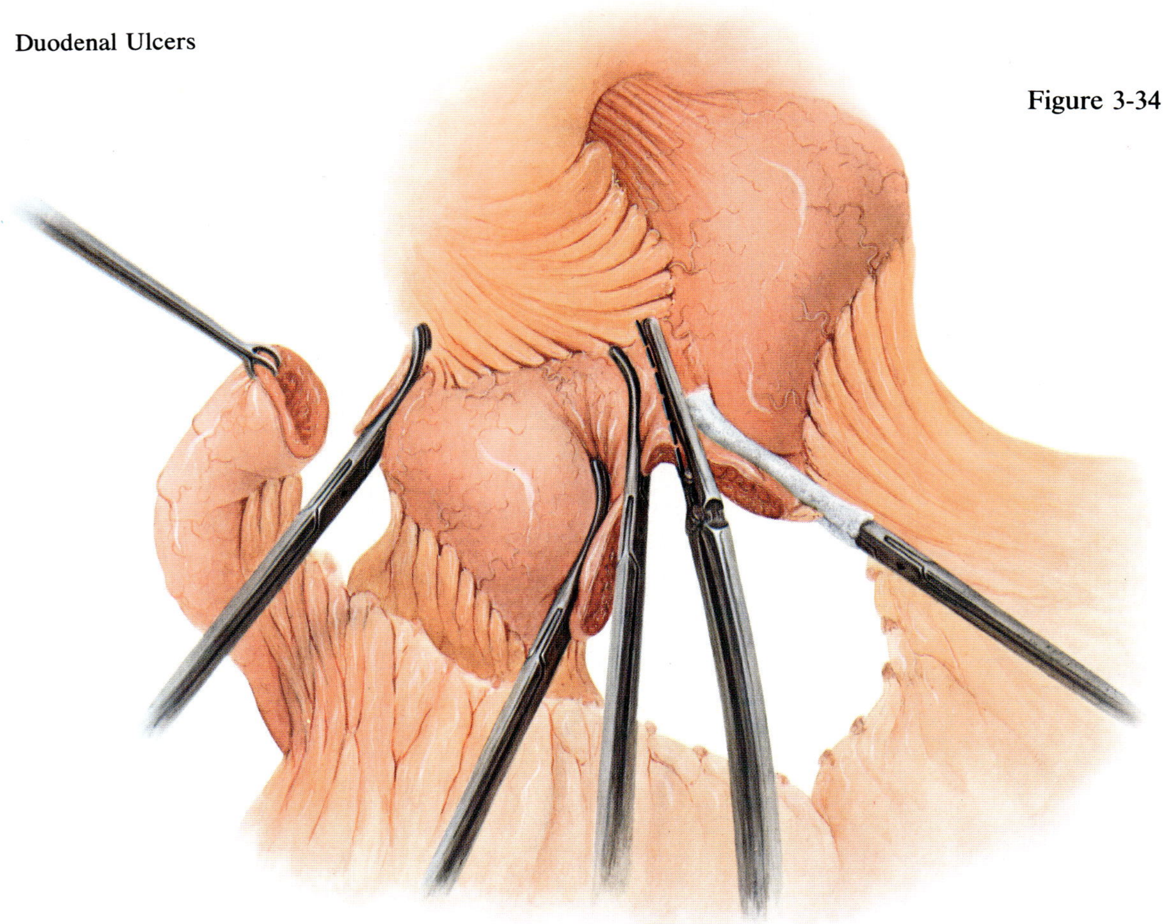

Figure 3-34

of nonabsorbable material (Fig. 3-35). Reconstruction by the performance of a gastroduodenostomy (Billroth I) is optional. The technique of anastomosis is highly individualized and varies from mechanical stapling to the traditional use of an inner layer of catgut and an outer layer of interrupted silk to the two-layer interrupted silk technique (Fig. 3-36). As with all anastomoses, five criteria should always be considered and fulfilled: (1) a good blood supply, (2) no tension, (3) an adequate lumen, (4) watertight construction, and (5) no distal obstruction.

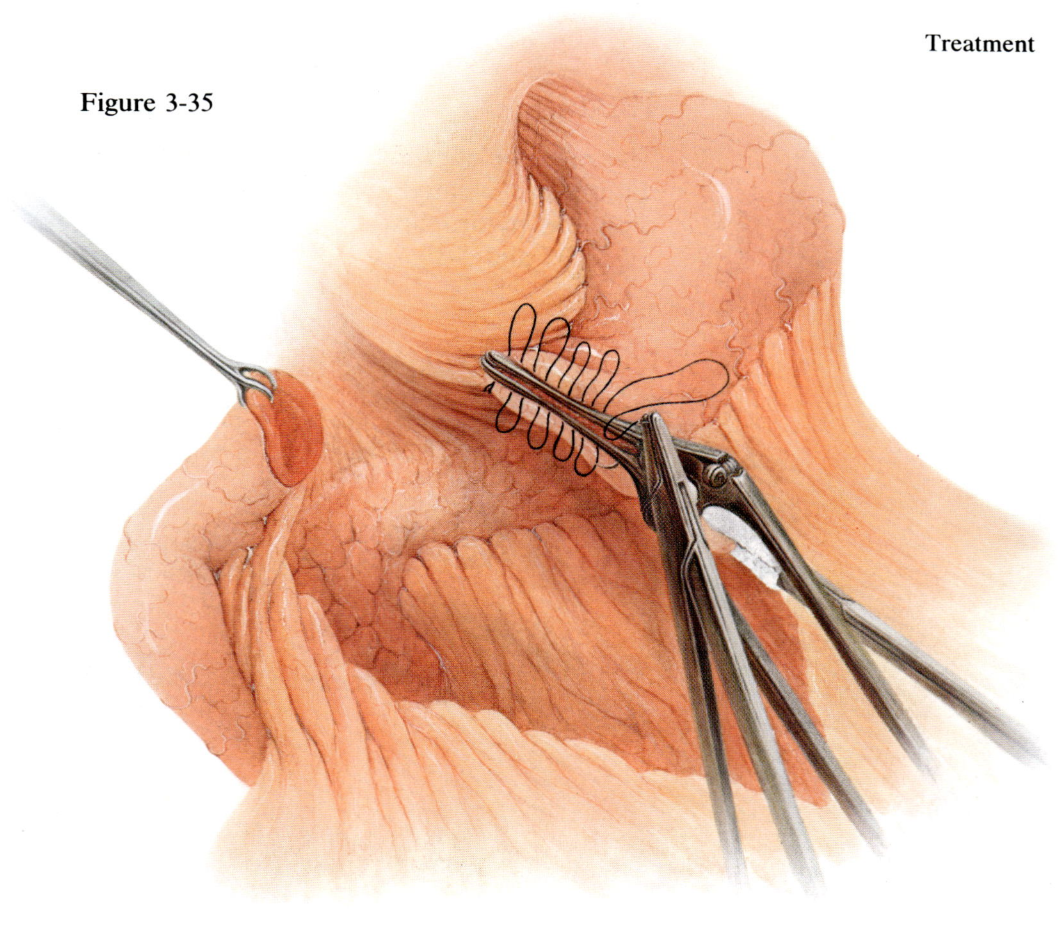

Figure 3-35

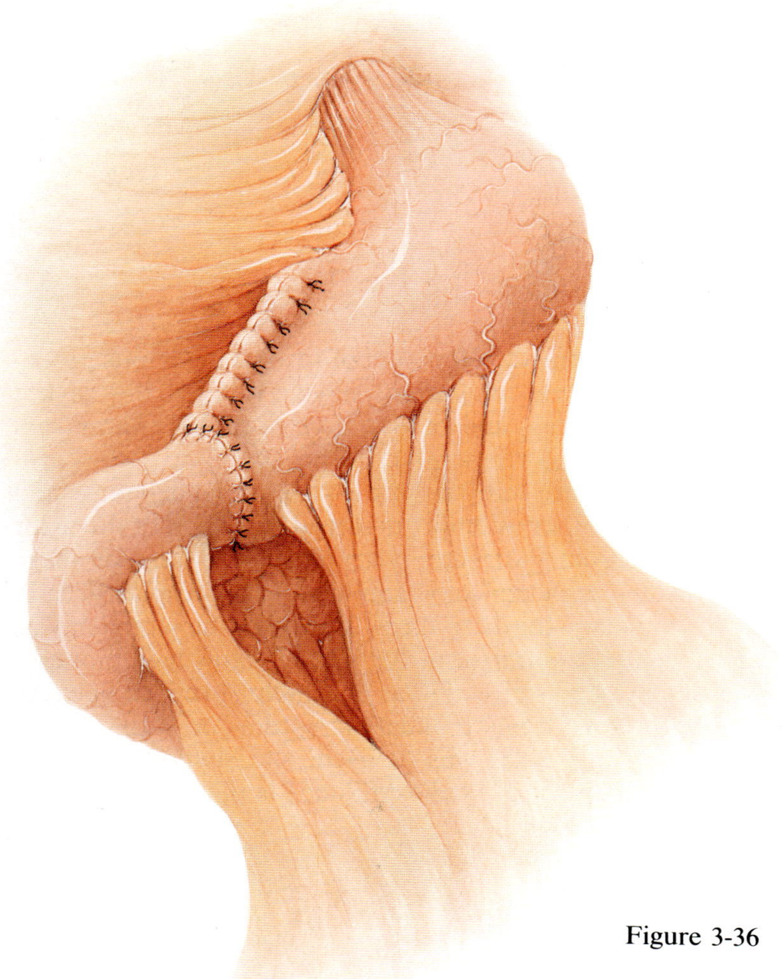

Figure 3-36

Results

The rates of operative mortality, recurrent ulceration, and diarrhea and dumping associated with truncal vagotomy and antrectomy, truncal vagotomy and pyloroplasty, and proximal gastric vagotomy are compared in Fig. 3-37 and 3-38.

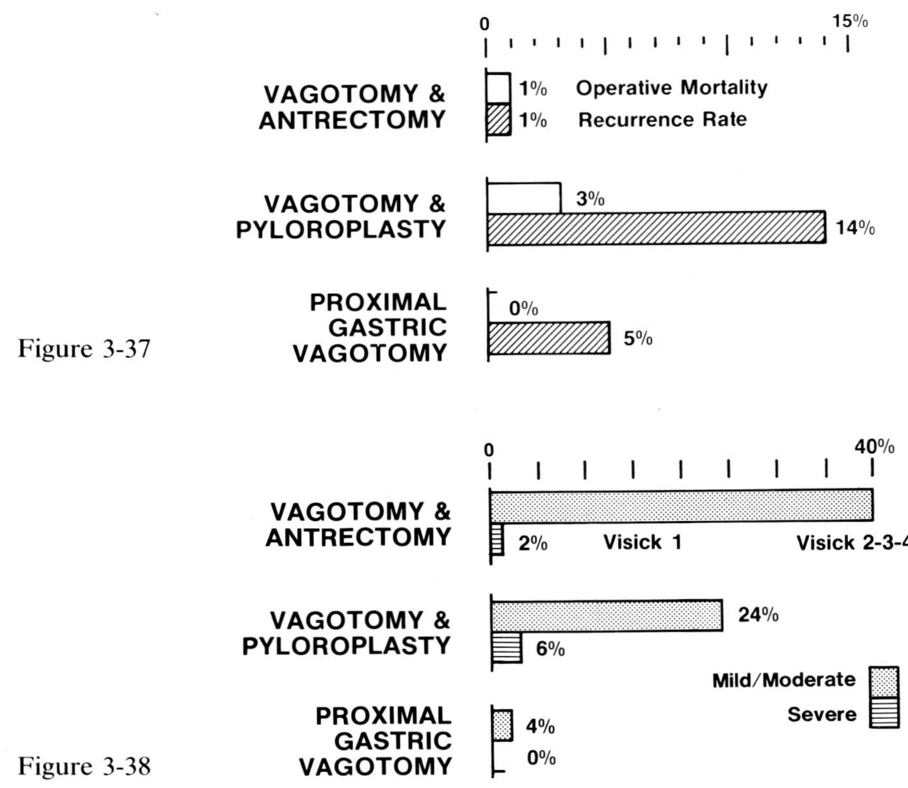

Figure 3-37

Figure 3-38

Historical Comment

Gastric surgery has promoted the development of several ingenious procedures (Fig. 3-39). Some of these operations have excluded the gastric antrum and resective procedures, and others have excluded the antrum and preserved the antral mucosa (Bancroft).

Serious attempts were made to reduce the gastric parietal cell mass and leave the ulcer in place, and other attempts involved resection of the ulcer in association with the partial gastrectomy (Fig. 3-40). Many of these procedures were associated with truncal vagotomy and pyloroplasty. Subtotal gastrectomy in which two-thirds to three-fourths of the stomach was removed enjoyed widespread enthusiasm for a time. However, none of these procedures proved to be as effective as originally surmised because of recurrent ulceration or severe postprandial symptoms or both.

Early on, pyloroplasty (Fig. 3-41) was devised, and several modifications were suggested. Perhaps the Heineke-Mikulicz is the simplest, easiest, and most effective approach.

Miscellaneous Gastric Operations

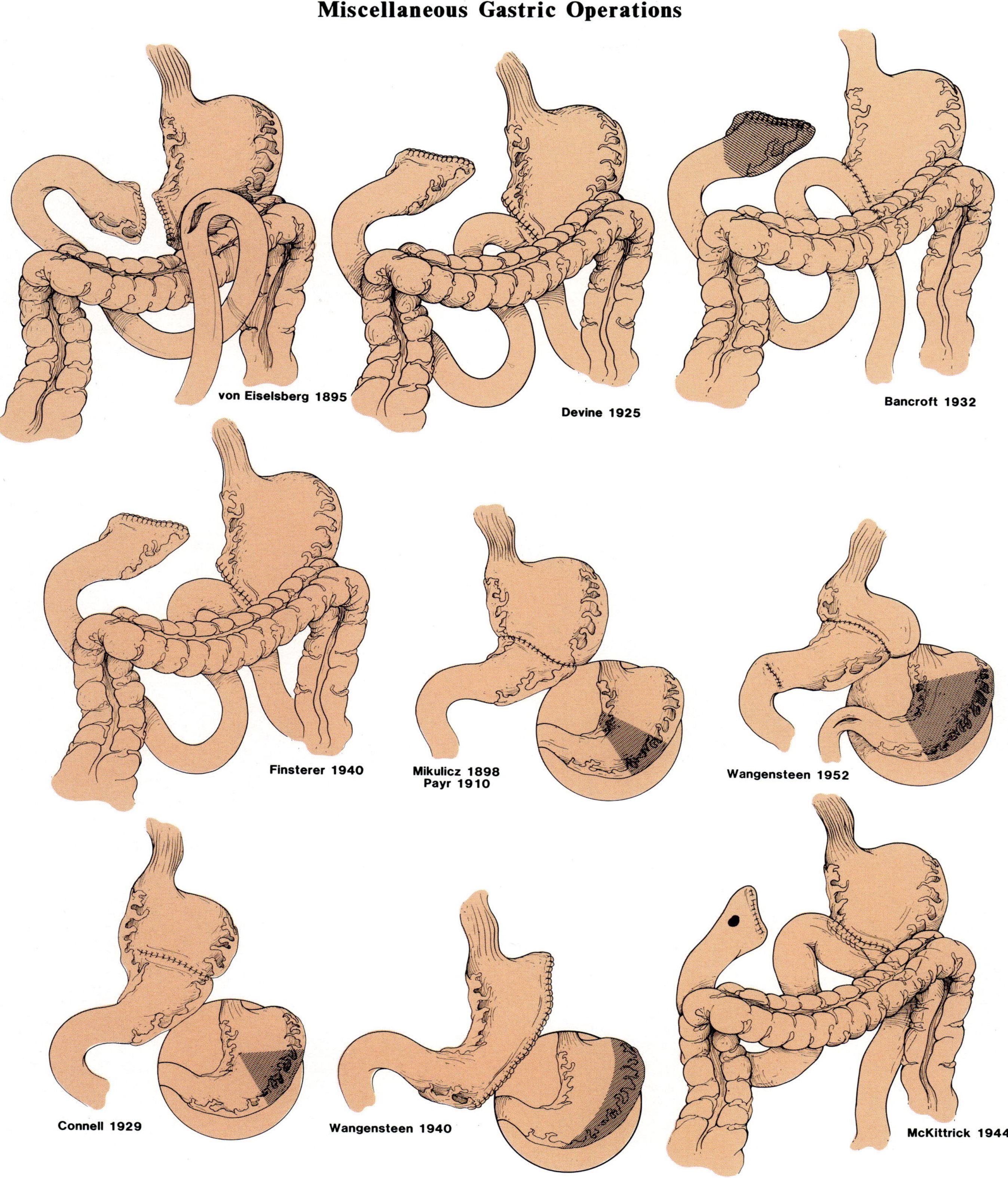

Figure 3-39

Duodenal Ulcer Procedures

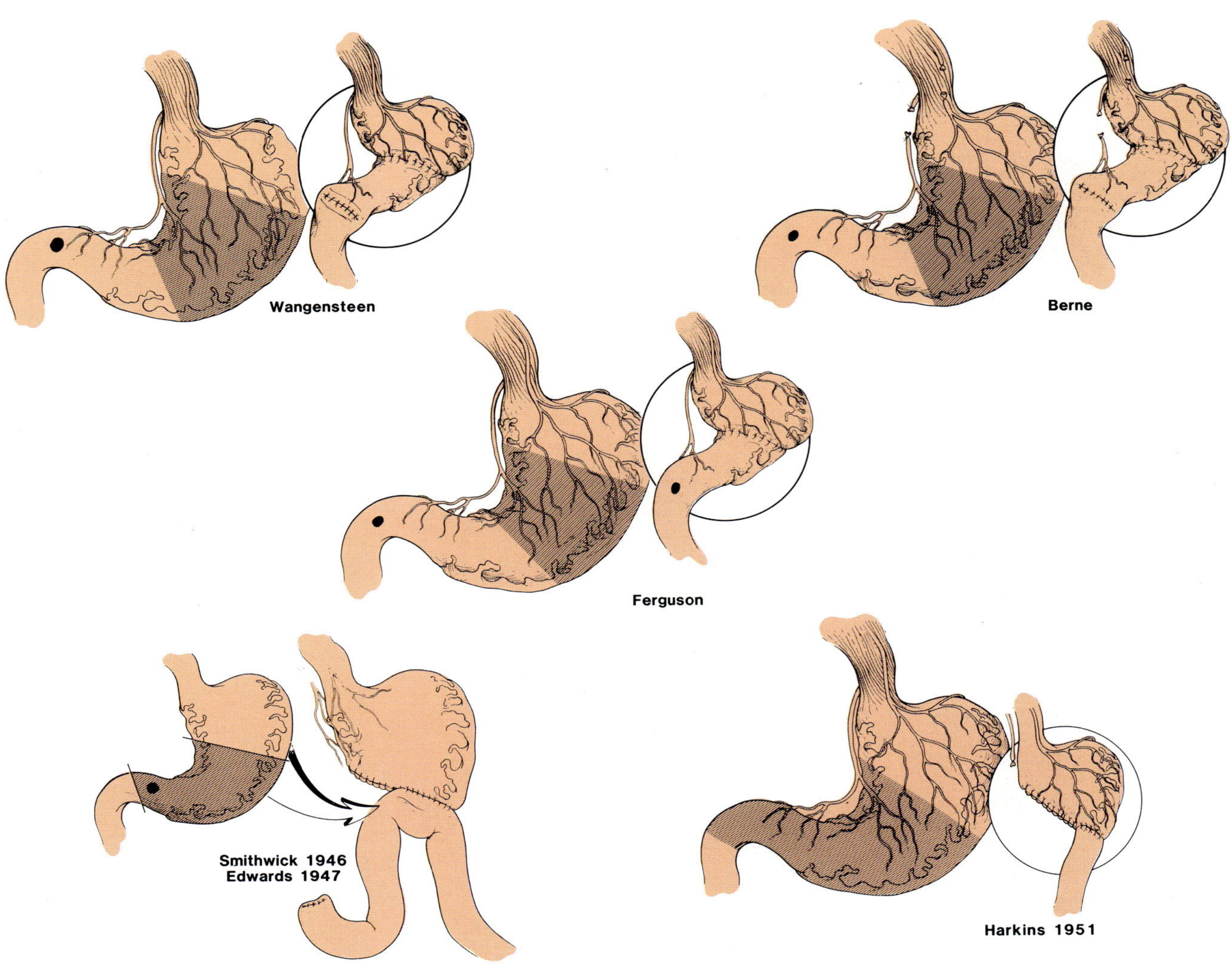

Figure 3-40

Pyloroplasty

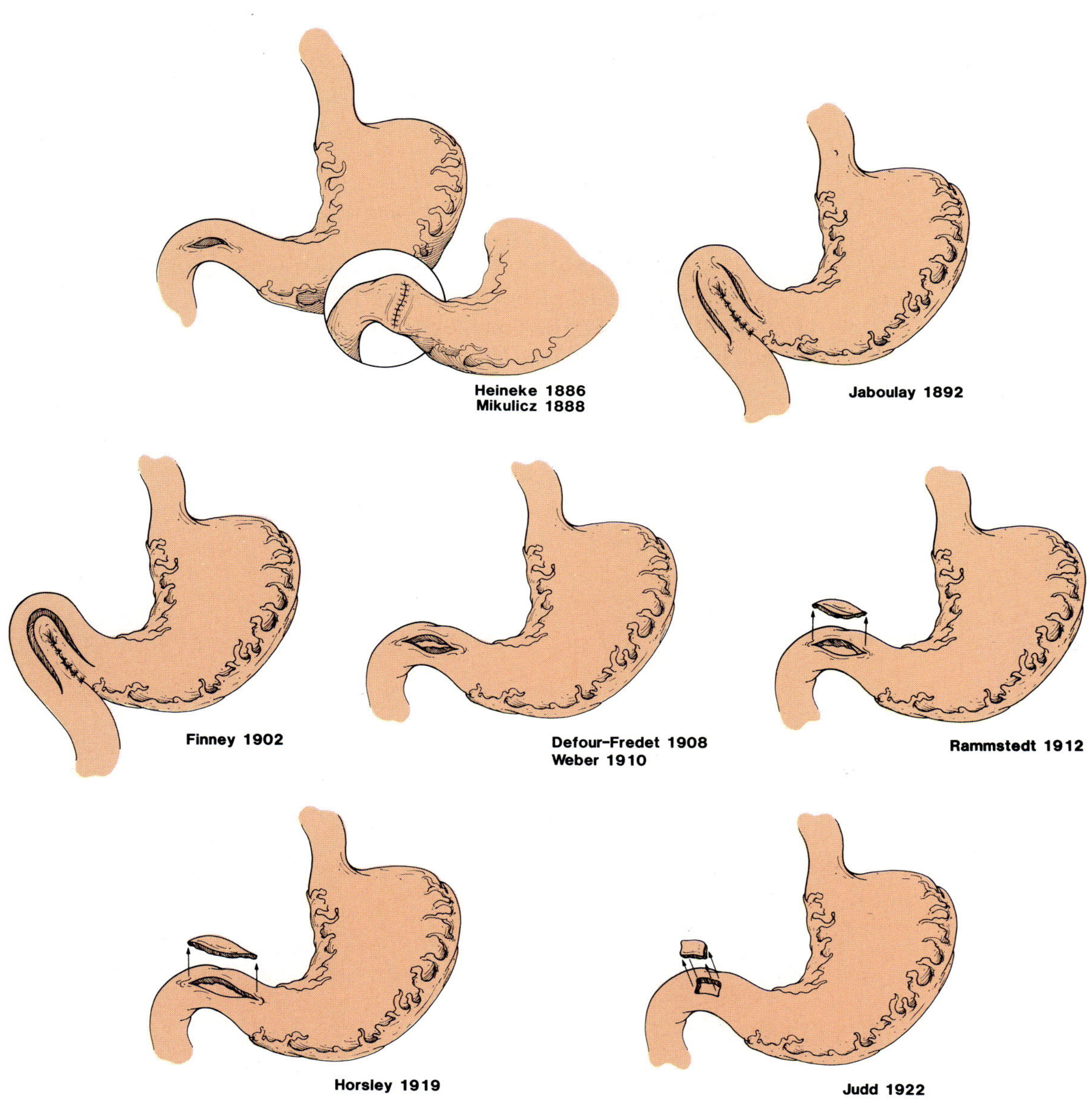

Figure 3-41

Suggested Reading

Duodenal Ulcers

1. Blackett RL, Johnston D (1981) Recurrent ulceration after highly selective vagotomy for duodenal ulcer. Br J Surg 68: 705
2. Christiansen J, Jensen H-E, Ejby-Poulsen P, et al (1981) Prospective controlled vagotomy trial for duodenal ulcer: primary results, sequelae, acid secretion, and recurrence rates two to five years after operation. Ann Surg 193: 49
3. Goligher JC (1974) A technique for highly selective (parietal cell or proximal gastric) vagotomy for duodenal ulcer. Br J Surg 61: 337
4. Goligher JC, Hill GL, Kenny TE, et al (1978) Proximal gastric vagotomy without drainage for duodenal ulcer: results after 5–8 years. Br J Surg 65: 145

5. Gorey TF, Lennon F, Heffernan SJ (1984) Highly selective vagotomy in duodenal ulceration and its complications: a 12-year review. Ann Surg 200: 181
6. Herrington JL Jr, Sawyers JL, Scott HW Jr (1973) A 25-year experience with vagotomy-antrectomy. Arch Surg 106: 469
7. Kennedy T, Johnston GW, Macrae KD, et al (1975) Proximal gastric vagotomy: interim results of a randomized controlled trial. Br Med J 2: 301
8. Knight CD Jr, van Heerden JA, Kelly KA (1983) Proximal gastric vagotomy—update. Ann Surg 197: 22
9. Stabile BE, Passaro E Jr (1984) Duodenal ulcer: a disease in evolution. Curr Probl Surg (January) 21: 1
10. Trout HH III (1982) Ulcer recurrence, morbidity, and mortality after operations for duodenal ulcer. Am J Surg 144: 570
11. Wylie CM (1981) The complex wane of peptic ulcer. II. Trends in duodenal and gastric ulcer admissions to 790 hospitals, 1974–1979. J Clin Gastroenterol 3: 333

Benign Gastric Lesions

4

Jon A. van Heerden

Stress Ulceration

Attention to stress ulceration was first popularized with the description of duodenal ulceration occurring in conjunction with lesions of the central nervous system (Cushing's ulcer) or in patients with massive burns (Curling's ulcer). The causes of this ulceration are, however, multifactorial; they include not only lesions of the central nervous system and burns but also sepsis of any cause or magnitude; hypotension; cardiac, hepatic, or renal failure; pulmonary insufficiency; and the administration of corticosteroids. Most stress ulcers are multiple, diffuse, and superficial.

The mainstay in the treatment of this entity is prevention. Prevention should concentrate on treatment of the inciting cause and the judicious use of antacids (the gastric pH should be maintained above 4.5). Treatment with antacids has proved superior to the H_2 blockers for prophylaxis of stress ulceration and has, in part, contributed to the markedly reduced incidence of gastroduodenal stress ulceration observed during the past decade.

Surgical intervention is indicated in approximately 10% of patients with stress ulceration. When indicated, however, surgical treatment should be radical. Lesser procedures such as vagotomy and pyloroplasty are thwarted by a high incidence of recurrent bleeding. The procedure of choice probably lies somewhere between vagotomy and pyloroplasty and total gastrectomy and has to be individualized according to the overall status of the patient, the risks involved, and the distribution of the ulceration. In particular, for stress ulcerations that involve the stomach, a near-total gastrectomy (about 95%) coupled with a truncal vagotomy and Roux-Y reconstruction (see Fig. 5-17), which eliminates bile reflux, might well be the surgical procedure of choice.

Chronic Benign Gastric Ulceration

Types of Chronic Gastric Ulcers

Chronic gastric ulcers are conveniently divided into three categories according to their anatomic site. Type I ulcers (Fig. 4-1) occur anywhere in the stomach except for the 2-cm area immediately proximal to the pylorus.

Figure 4-1

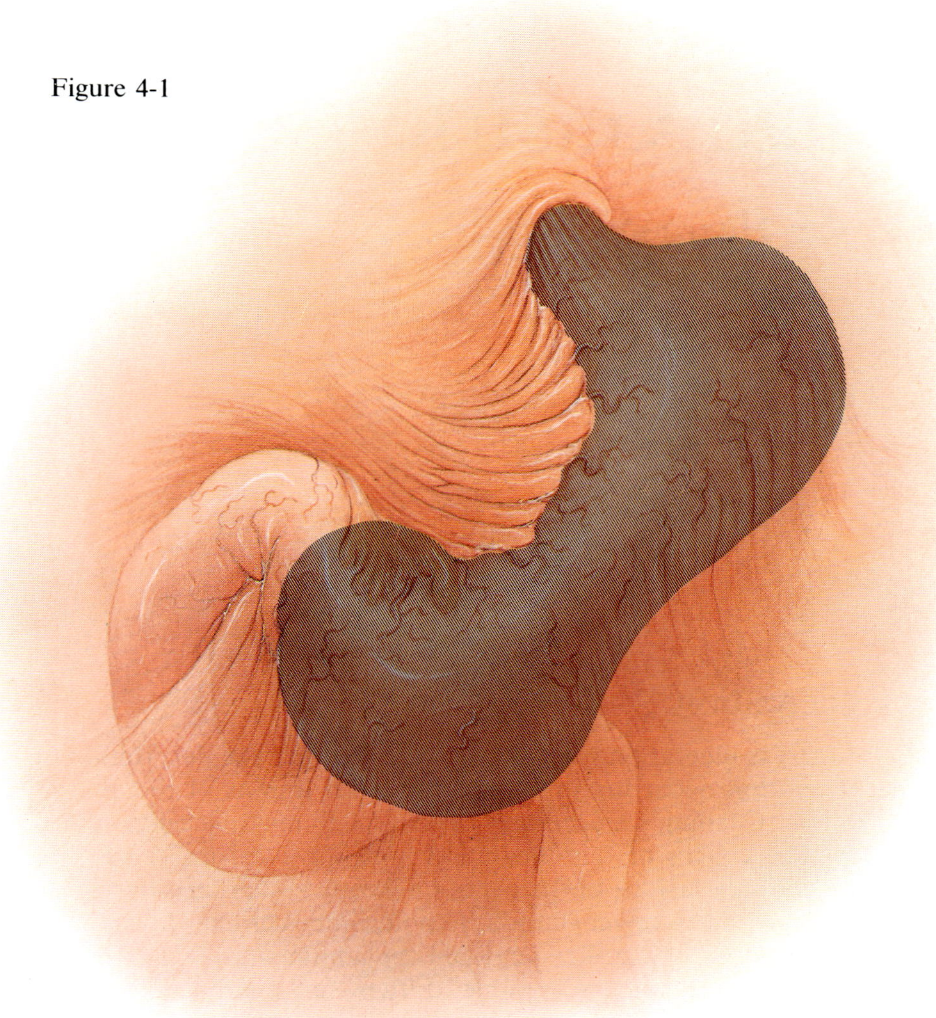

Type II ulcers (Fig. 4-2) are type I ulcers that occur in conjunction with a duodenal ulcer. As is true for type I ulcers, type II lesions have no ulceration in the 2-cm zone proximal to the pylorus. Type III ulcers (Fig. 4-3) are located in the 2-cm zone proximal to the pylorus. They are often termed "prepyloric" gastric ulcers. The importance of these categories lies in the possible etiologic differences and thus the subsequent differences in surgical therapy.

Figure 4-2

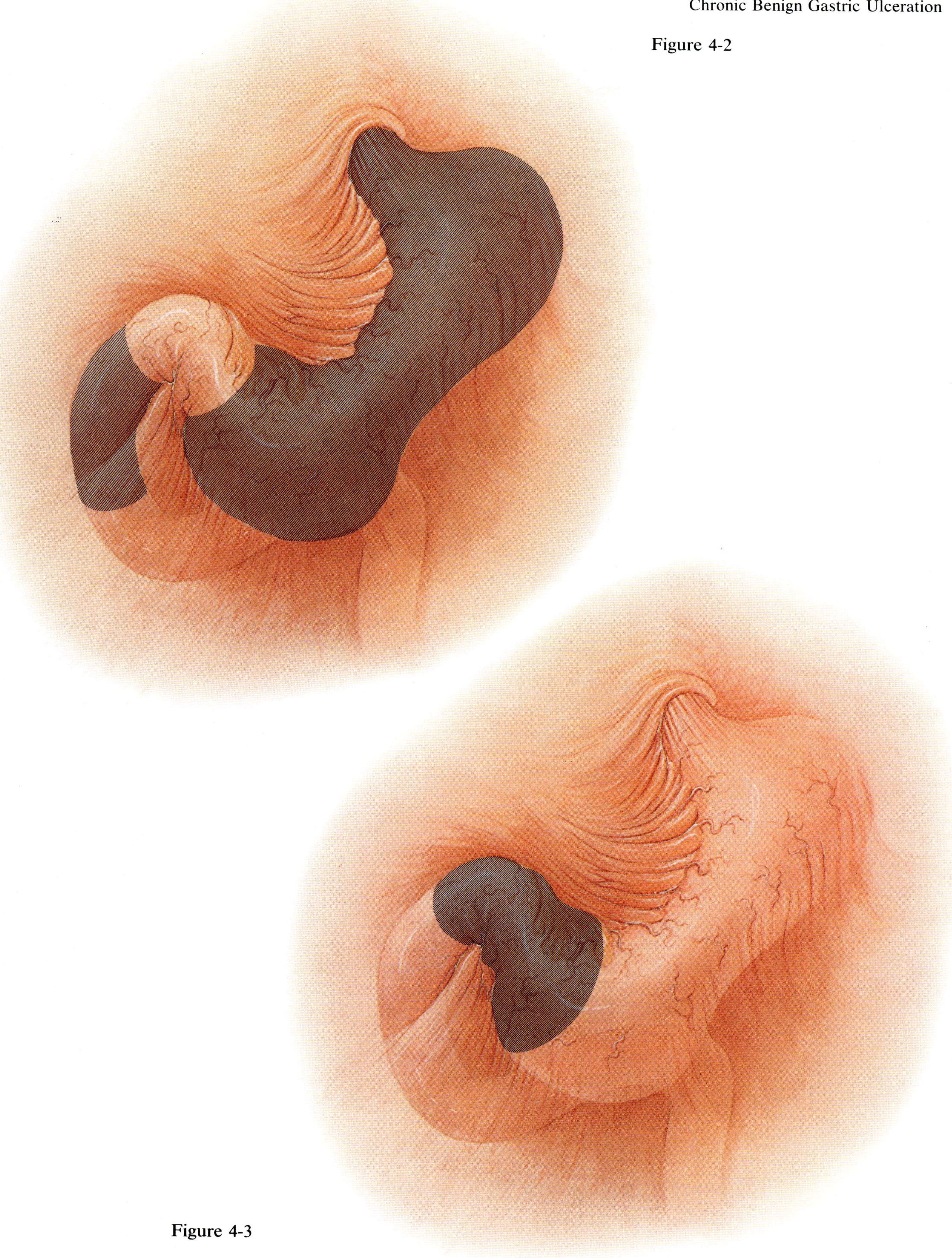

Figure 4-3

Etiology

The cause of chronic gastric ulceration is multifactorial and complex. The etiologic theories to be discussed are inexact, and the true cause is probably a combination of any, or all, of these factors.

Antral Stasis (Dragstedt) (Fig. 4-4). According to this theory, antral stasis results in increased secretion of gastrin by the antral G cells, which in turn leads to increased secretion of hydrochloric acid by the parietal cell mass, and gastric ulceration ensues. The "hole" in this theory is that hypersecretion is seldom found in type I gastric ulceration with conventional methods of analysis.

Gastric Mucosal Barrier and Back Diffusion (Davenport) (Fig. 4-5). This theory states that, for reasons that are as yet unclear, the pylorus is, or becomes, incompetent and allows reflux of duodenal contents into the stomach. This reflux, in turn, causes changes in both the quantity and the quality of the gastric mucosal barrier (gastric mucus); the result is back diffusion of both hydrochloric acid and pepsinogen into the gastric mucosal cells and subsequent disruption and gastric ulceration.

Junctional "Weakness" (Oi) (Fig. 4-6). Oi stated that a locus minoris resistentiae exists at the line where the antral epithelium meets the epithelium of the corpus of the stomach. This junctional area coincides with the angularis of the stomach, where most type I gastric ulcers occur.

Gastritis (Lawson) (Fig. 4-7). For many years, Lawson has presented excellent basic data to substantiate the presence of an abnormal mucosa in patients with gastric ulceration. This abnormal mucosa is thought to be secondary, once again, to reflux caused by an incompetent pylorus. He has emphasized that this abnormal mucosa should be removed (that is, resected) during most operations for chronic gastric ulceration.

Treatment

Because of the diverse causes of chronic gastric ulceration, surgical therapy has similarly been extremely varied. The methods range from simple excision (which is associated with a high recurrence rate) to resective procedures with or without vagotomy. Within the past decade, excision of the ulcer coupled with proximal gastric vagotomy has become a well-accepted approach; the results, however, have been disappointing. The cause of type III ulcers seems to be similar to that of duodenal ulcers (that is, hypersecretion), and treatment of these ulcers is directed toward acid reduction (proximal gastric vagotomy or truncal vagotomy and antrectomy). Type I ulcers are best treated with a distal gastrectomy and gastroduodenostomy without vagotomy, and treatment of type II ulcers should be similar but should also include either a total gastric or a truncal vagotomy. For all gastric ulcers, regardless of site, a thorough biopsy is indicated to rule out gastric malignant disease.

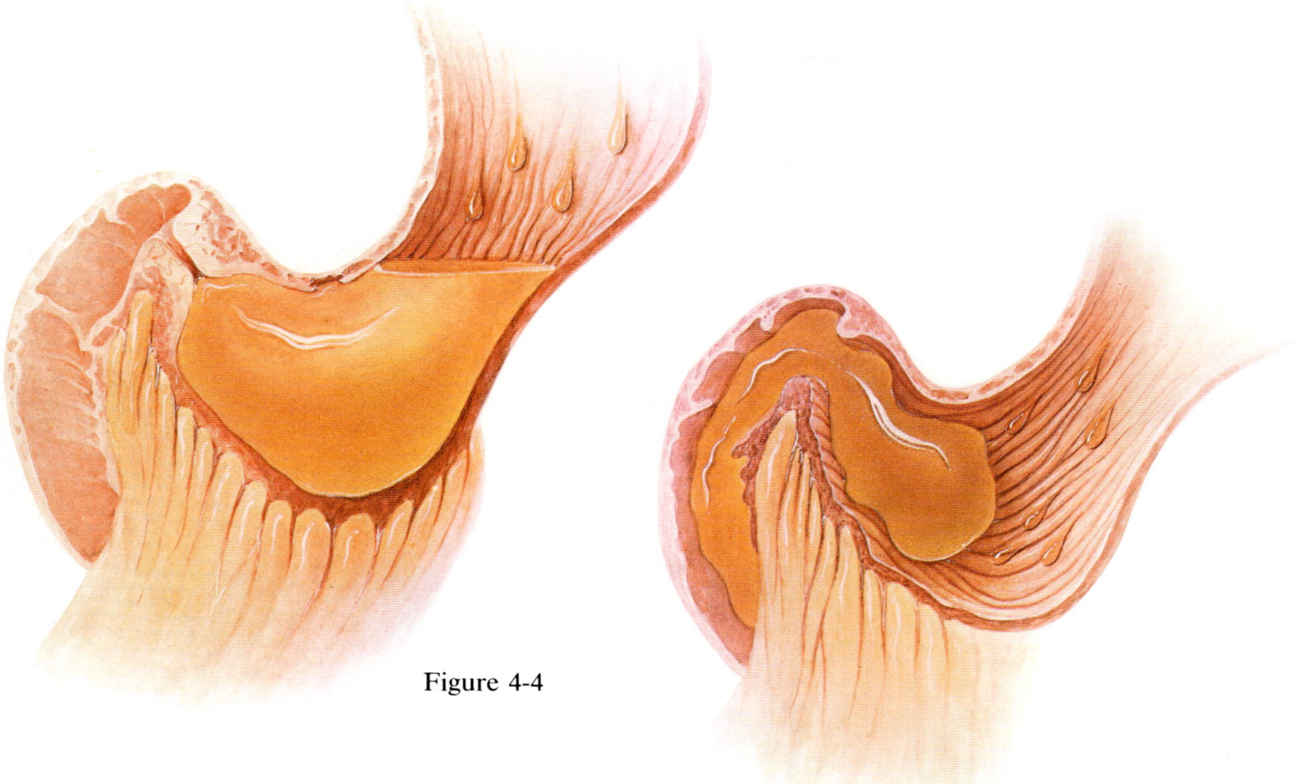

Figure 4-4

Figure 4-5

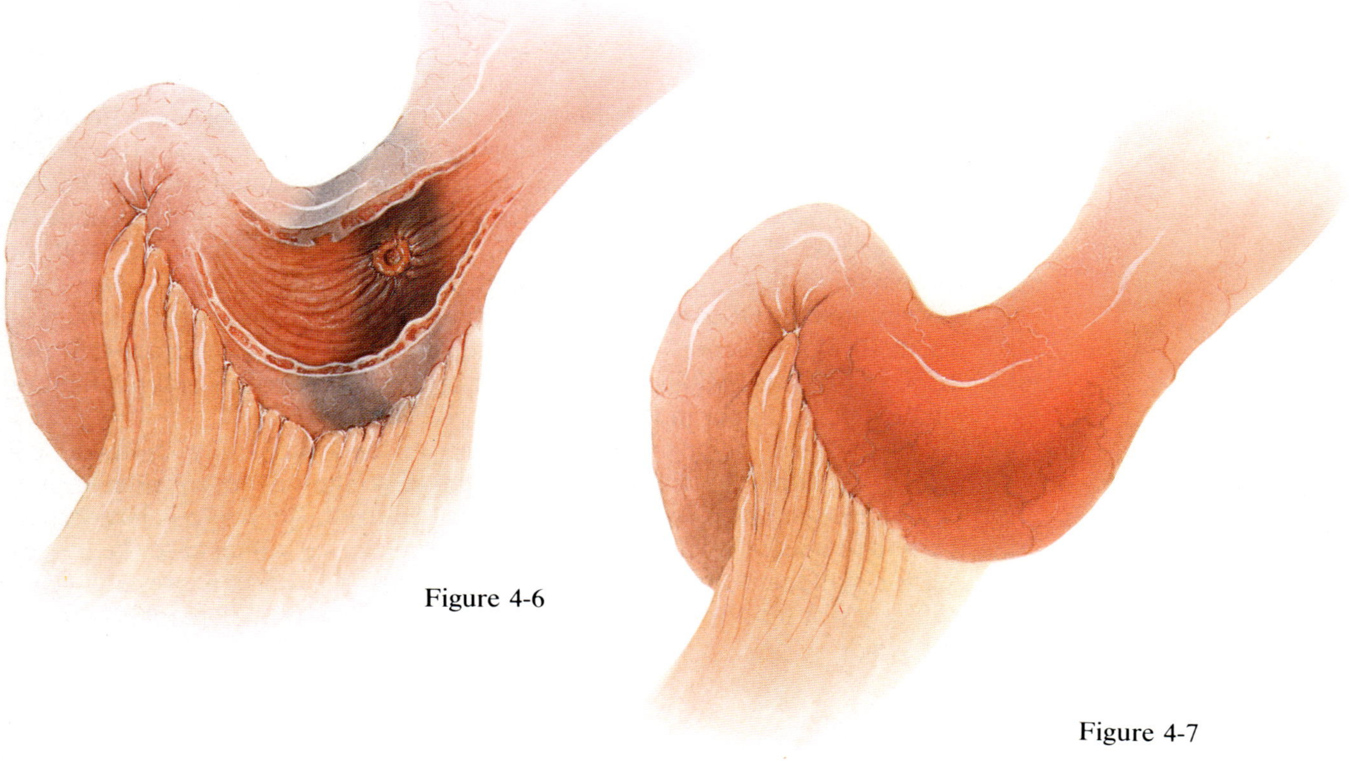

Figure 4-6

Figure 4-7

Figure 4-8

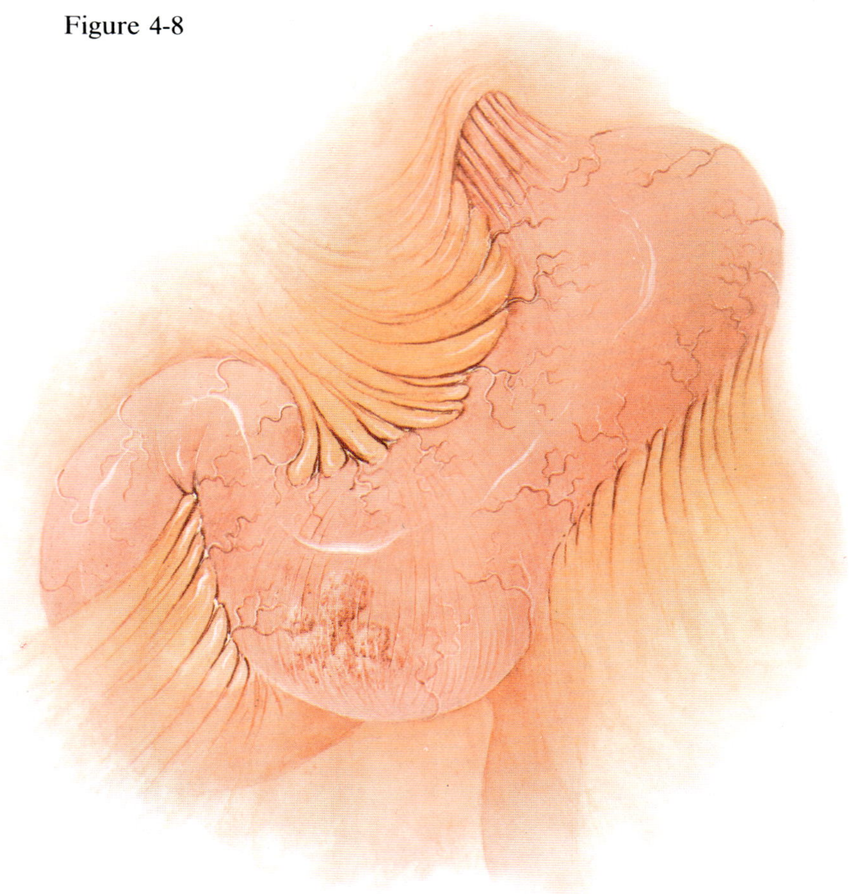

Gastric Polyps

Gastric polyps are quite rare—they occur in approximately 0.4% to 0.7% of the general population. Pathologically, gastric polyps may conveniently be divided into three types: (1) epithelial (adenomatous or hyperplastic), the most common type; (2) mesenchymal (leiomyomas, fibromas, lipomas, neurogenic tumors, and vascular tumors); and (3) miscellaneous (carcinoid tumors, heterotopic pancreas, and hamartomas associated with the Peutz-Jeghers syndrome). Epithelial (adenomatous) polyps are of most interest to surgeons. These polyps may be single (Fig. 4-8), multiple (Fig. 4-9), or diffuse (so-called *polypeux en nappe*) (Fig. 4-10). Most gastric polyps are asymptomatic. Of concern are the potentials for bleeding, which occurs in about 10% of patients, and malignant degeneration, which occurs in about 2.5% of patients. Malignant change is seldom observed in polyps that are smaller than 2.0 cm in diameter.

Most gastric polyps are easily removed endoscopically. Surgical removal by either gastrectomy or gastrotomy should be considered if a patient is symptomatic, hemorrhage has occurred, the polyp is larger than 2 cm in diameter, gastric achlorhydria is present (in which case the potential for malignant disease is higher), or diffuse polyposis is present—particularly if a family history of gastric polyposis with malignant change is elicited.

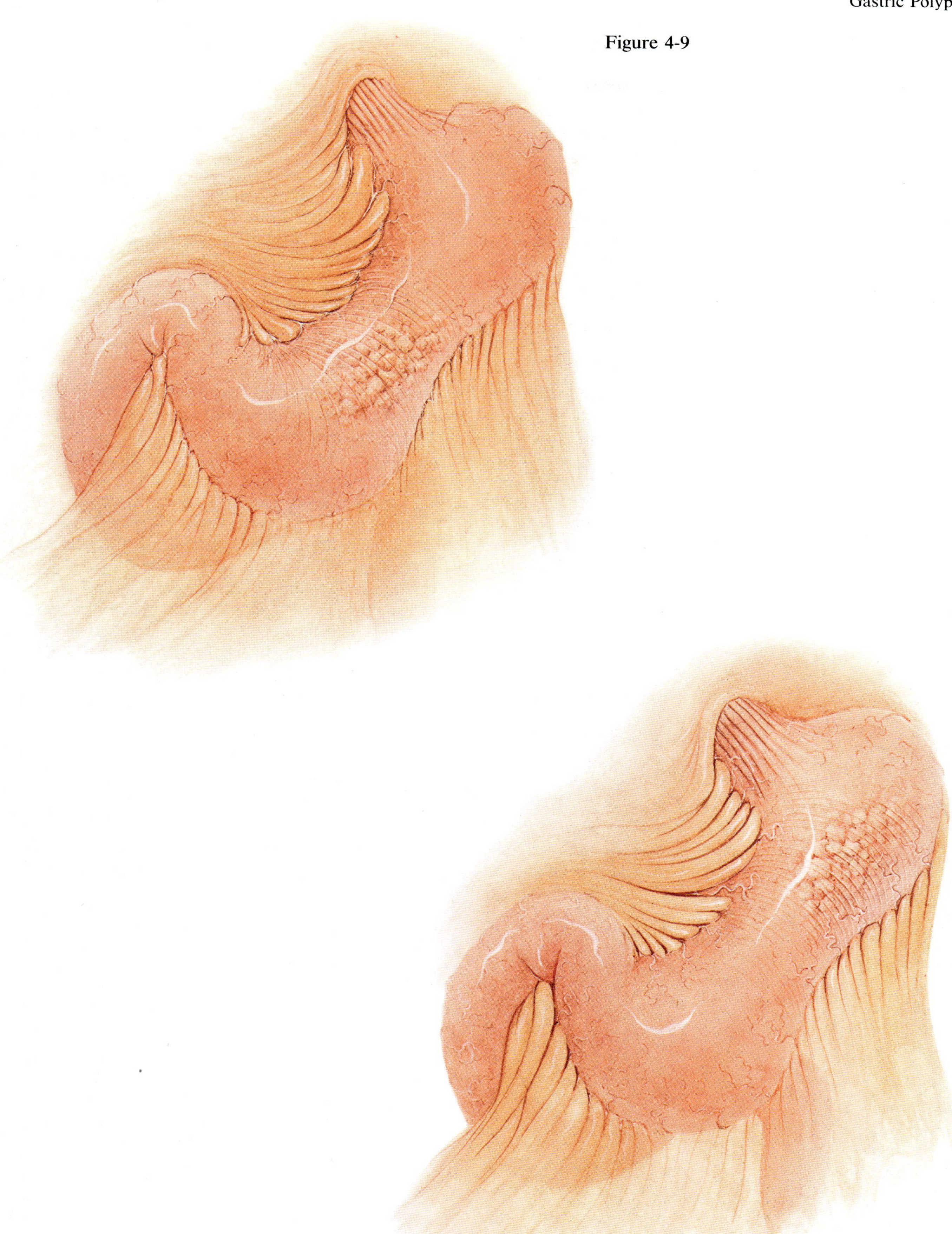

Figure 4-9

Figure 4-10

Suggested Reading

Stress Ulceration

1. Halloran LG, Zfass AM, Gayle WE, et al (1980) Prevention of acute gastrointestinal complications after severe head injury: a controlled trial of cimetidine prophylaxis. Am J Surg 139: 44
2. Hastings PR, Skillman JJ, Bushnell LS, et al (1978) Antacid titration in the prevention of acute gastrointestinal bleeding: a controlled, randomized trial in 100 critically ill patients. N Engl J Med 298: 1041
3. Hubert JP Jr., Kiernan PD, Welch JS, et al (1980) The surgical management of bleeding stress ulcers. Ann Surg 191: 672
4. Zinner MJ, Zuidema GD, Smith PL, et al (1981) The prevention of upper gastrointestinal tract bleeding in patients in an intensive care unit. Surg Gynecol Obstet 153: 214

Gastric Ulcers

1. Adami H-O, Enander LK, Enskog L, et al (1984) Recurrences 1 to 10 years after highly selective vagotomy in prepyloric and duodenal ulcer disease: frequency, pattern, and predictors. Ann Surg 199: 393
2. Davis Z, Verheyden CN, van Heerden JA, et al (1977) The surgically treated chronic gastric ulcer: an extended followup. Ann Surg 185: 205
3. Emås S, Hammarberg C (1983) Prospective, randomized trial of selective proximal vagotomy with ulcer excision and partial gastrectomy with gastroduodenostomy in the treatment of corporeal gastric ulcer. Am J Surg 146: 631
4. Jensen HE, Kjaergaard J, Meisner S (1983) Ulcer recurrence two to twelve years after parietal cell vagotomy for duodenal ulcer. Surgery 94: 802
5. Jordan PH Jr. (1981) Treatment of gastric ulcer by parietal cell vagotomy and excision of the ulcer: rationale and early results. Arch Surg 116: 1320
6. Reid DA, Duthie HL, Bransom CJ, et al (1982) Late follow-up of highly selective vagotomy with excision of the ulcer compared with Billroth I gastrectomy for treatment of benign gastric ulcer. Br J Surg 69: 605

Gastric Polyps

1. Bone GE, McClelland RN (1976) Management of gastric polyps—a review. Rev Surg 33: 211
2. King RM, van Heerden JA, Weiland LH (1982) The management of gastric polyps. Surg Gynecol Obstet 155: 846
3. Monaco AP, Roth SI, Castleman B, et al (1962) Adenomatous polyps of the stomach: a clinical and pathological study of 153 cases. Cancer 15: 456

Malignant Gastric Lesions

5

William H. ReMine

In recent years, important advances have been made in the early diagnosis of cancer of the stomach, although a low index of suspicion often vitiates this advantage.

When an alleged ''benign'' gastric ulcer persists for a prolonged time (2 to 3 months), exploration is indicated because medical management of benign gastric ulcer is only partially satisfactory.[5]

Once gastric malignant disease has been diagnosed, operation should follow shortly. The importance of exploration must be fully realized because without operation there is no known cure.

Partial or Subtotal Gastrectomy

The abdomen may be entered in several ways, and each approach has a large and enthusiastic group of supporters. Instead of the use of a ''routine'' incision, the type of incision used should be based on the particular physical build of a patient. Whether a transverse, oblique, or vertical incision is used depends on the conditions at hand.

After the abdomen is opened, it should be carefully explored to determine the presence or absence of metastatic lesions or extension to other structures. Radical procedures should not be performed for palliation.

When the lesion is confined to the stomach, or perhaps has extended only to the regional lymph nodes, an operation with the hope of cure is performed. Currently, two procedures are primarily available to the surgeon, and the choice depends on the location of the lesion.

If the lesion is in the distal half of the stomach, it is our policy to perform a radical subtotal gastrectomy. This procedure embodies most of the features of an effective operation for cancer and is directed toward the eradication of all possible areas of spread. The lesion is removed en bloc with the entire omentum, about 80% to 85% of the stomach, the spleen and its hilar lymph nodes, the first portion of the duodenum, and all associated lymph nodes around the head of the pancreas. In addition, the node-bearing tissue from the duodenohepatic pedicle and the gastrohepatic omentum is removed with the lesion. The entire lesser curvature of the stomach and all of the lymph nodes along it are removed by means of a Hofmeister-Polya resection. An end-to-side anastomosis between the gastric remnant and the first portion of the jejunum reestablishes gastrointestinal continuity.

Figure 5-1

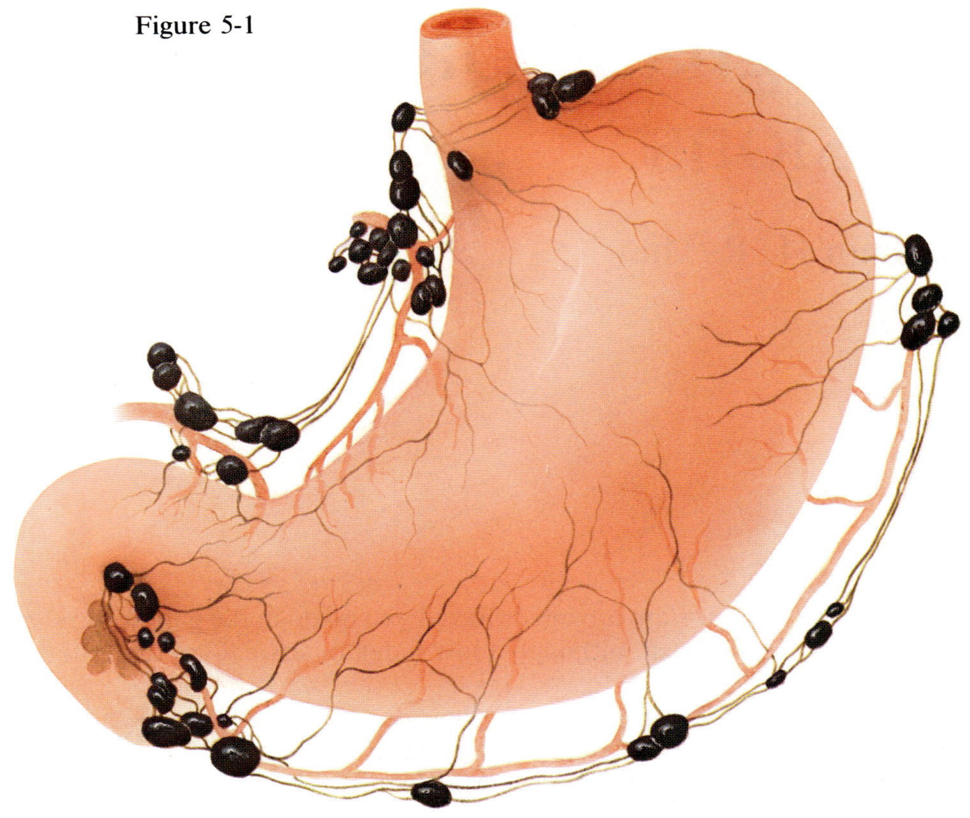

If the lesion is in the middle or upper third of the stomach, total gastrectomy with removal of the previously mentioned areas of possible spread to adjacent lymph nodes becomes necessary. Continuity is reestablished by means of an esophagojejunostomy in an end-to-end manner, preferably a Hunt type (see Fig. 5-21). If the lesion can be completely removed by subtotal gastric resection, then at least a portion of the stomach is left attached to the esophagus, and the procedure is carried out in this manner.

An effective operation for cancer entails removal of all of the greater omentum and all areas of regional lymphatic drainage when possible. In the past, the spleen has not always been removed when the lesion involved only the distal portion of the stomach; evidence suggests, however, that removal is advisable.[4] For this reason, we have recently tended to remove the spleen regardless of the location of a gastric lesion, even if it is in the distal portion of the stomach. If a lesion is in the proximal portion of the stomach, the spleen is removed routinely. Total gastrectomy, which always includes splenectomy, is reserved for patients in whom all areas of malignant involvement cannot be removed with subtotal gastrectomy.

Perhaps the most important advancement in the treatment of carcinoma of the stomach is proper consideration of the lymph nodes. The reports of Delamere et al.,[3] Rouvière,[8] and Coller et al.[2] indicate that 11 groups of lymph nodes are of great importance (Fig. 5-1): lower coronary, upper coronary, right paracardial, left paracardial, posterior paracardial, splenic, right gastroepiploic, subpyloric, suprapyloric, suprápancreatic, and celiac. All of these groups should be considered for the performance of a total gastrectomy, whereas the splenic, right gastroepiploic, subpyloric, suprapyloric, suprapancreatic, and celiac lymph nodes are of utmost importance for radical subtotal gastric resection.

Figure 5-2

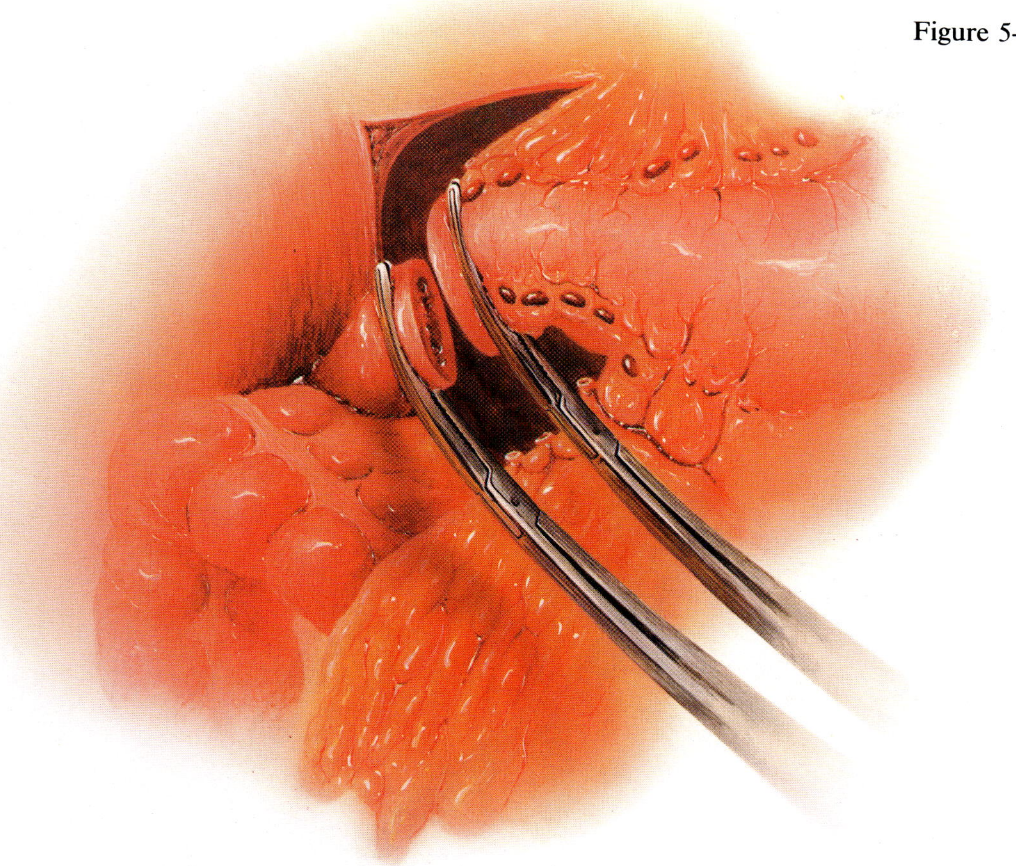

Billroth I Procedure

The Billroth I procedure (Fig. 5-2)[1] is seldom used in the surgical treatment of gastric carcinoma. Most commonly, the size and location of the lesion render a gastroduodenal anastomosis unsatisfactory if one hopes to remove all possible areas of local spread (including the subpyloric nodes and the proximal portion of the duodenum) and perform an effective operation for cancer. Such an anastomosis is especially contraindicated if the patient is obese and the duodenum is deeply situated. This type of procedure may be associated with a tendency to remove too small a portion of the stomach; in such cases, a patient's chances for survival are compromised because of inadequate resection. Incomplete removal is especially likely in the presence of a high-grade malignant or scirrhous lesion that tends to spread intramurally along the gastric wall.

In rare cases, a small, early growth in the prepyloric antrum that shows no evidence of spread either to lymph nodes or by direct extension can be resected and gastrointestinal continuity can be reestablished with the Billroth I procedure.

When the Billroth I procedure is used (Fig. 5-3), the Schoemaker-Billroth I method (Fig. 5-4) has proved to be particularly useful.

Figure 5-3

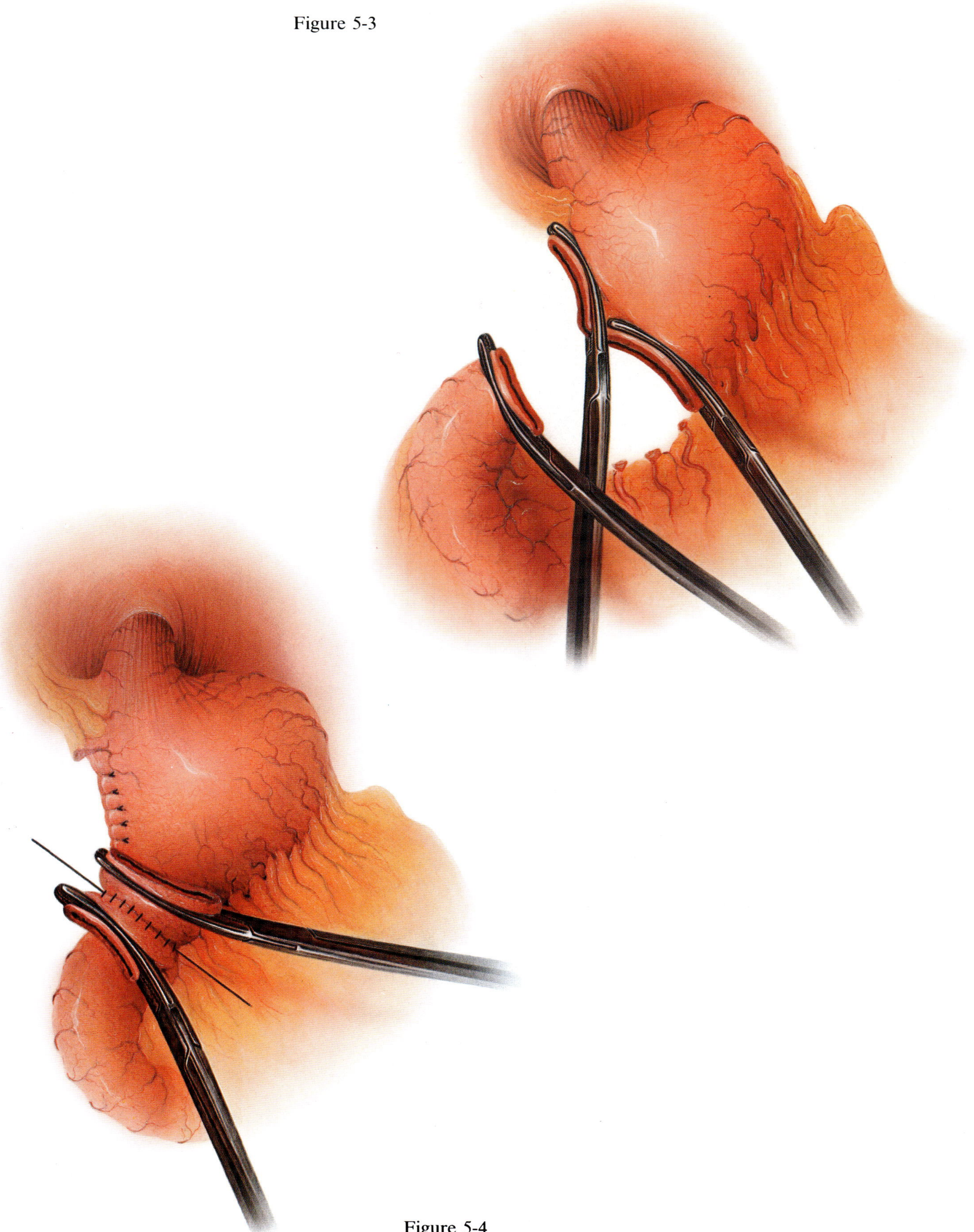

Figure 5-4

Figure 5-5

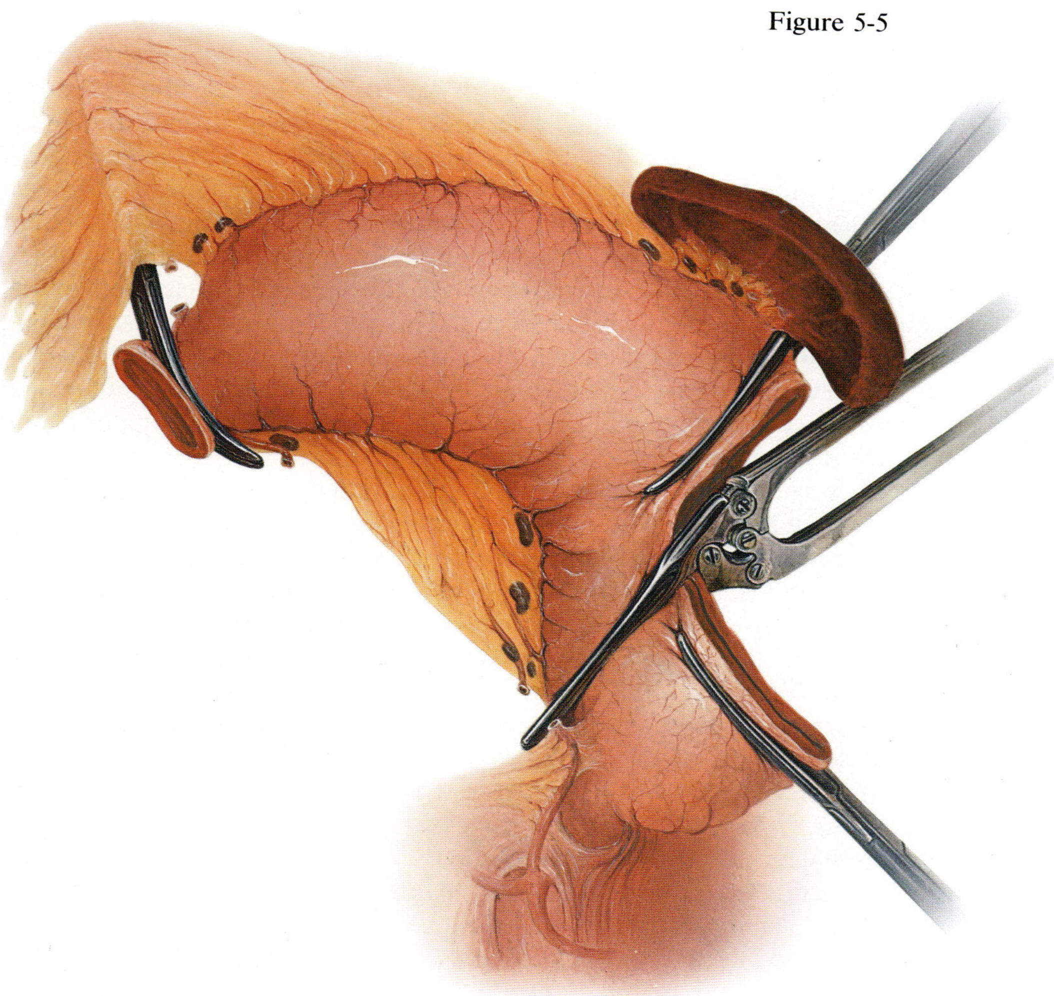

Radical Subtotal Gastrectomy

Dissection is started at the splenic flexure of the colon and progresses toward the hepatic flexure, and the entire omentum is dissected free from the colon and left attached to the greater curvature of the stomach. The duodenum is then ''kocherized'' to free it up so that adequate dissection around the head of the pancreas and first portion of the duodenum can be performed. All of the lymph node-bearing tissue around the head of the pancreas is then dissected out en bloc but is left attached to the duodenum to be removed with it. This procedure is particularly important for the subpyloric nodes.[6] Superiorly, the node-bearing tissue in the duodenohepatic pedicle and any associated lymph nodes are dissected out, and they, too, are left attached to the duodenum. The duodenum is then dissected down to a point proximal to the common duct, where it is transected (Fig. 5-2). If the surgeon is uncertain about the integrity of the common duct, a long-limbed T-tube may be inserted into the common duct with the long limb extending down into the second or third portion of the duodenum. The duodenal stump is closed with two rows of continuous absorbable sutures and an outer row of fine-silk sutures.

The stomach is then elevated, and the dissection is continued laterally (Fig. 5-5) across the superior margin of the pancreas, and all node-bearing tissue around the common hepatic artery is removed. This dissection is continued to the celiac axis (Fig. 5-5), where the celiac nodes are dissected out carefully and the left gastric artery is ligated, leaving the ascending branch to the gastric remnant. The node-bearing tissue around the celiac axis is carefully removed with the stomach en bloc. The spleen is left attached to the greater curvature of the stomach by the short gastric vessels (vasa brevia) and the splenic artery, and the splenic veins are secured with two ligatures of heavy silk. Occasionally, a portion of the tail of the pancreas may have to be removed with the spleen to resect all of the lymph nodes in the hilus of the spleen. This procedure is necessary when the tail of the pancreas is intimately associated with the splenic hilus. In such cases, care must be taken to ligate the pancreatic duct with silk ligatures because any leakage could readily digest absorbable material and produce a pancreatic fistula.

Occasionally, a lesion may involve the transverse mesocolon or the transverse colon by seeding or direct extension. When this occurs, these areas are removed with the resected portion of the stomach.

At this point, the stomach should be well mobilized to allow an adequate resection that involves removal of approximately 80% to 85% of the stomach and all of the tissue on the lesser curvature (Fig. 5-5).

The site for transection of the stomach is carefully selected, and two large, curved forceps are applied at the greater curvature. These will determine the size of the proposed gastrojejunal stoma. After the tissue between these two clamps has been severed with a scalpel, a Payr clamp is placed (Fig. 5-5) such that the entire lesser curvature of the stomach up to the esophagus may be removed with the resected specimen and all its associated node-bearing tissue. Great care must be taken to preserve the ascending branch of the left gastric artery; this precaution ensures an adequate blood supply to the gastric remnant. Another large, curved forceps is placed next to the Payr clamp; they are then separated with a scalpel, and the specimen is removed.

The lesser curvature is closed by undersewing the Payr clamp with a row of continuous fine absorbable sutures, the clamp is then removed, and the first row of sutures is oversewn with another row of continuous fine absorbable sutures. Finally, the entire area is turned in with a row of carefully placed, interrupted silk mattress sutures.

For partial or subtotal gastrectomy, we generally prefer the Hofmeister-Polya anastomosis (Fig. 5-6 and 5-7)—attachment of the distal limb of the jejunum to the greater curvature of the stomach. In recent years, this anastomosis has been used for most patients who have undergone partial gastrectomy at the Mayo Clinic. When high subtotal gastrectomy is performed, a posterior anastomosis may not be feasible, and the jejunal loops are then brought anterior to the transverse colon. The relationship to the colon (anterior or posterior) is the surgeon's choice.

The Hofmeister-Polya end-to-side anastomosis is constructed to the first portion of the jejunum (Fig. 5-7) with the shortest possible loop of jejunum. This goal is accomplished with an outer (or seromuscular) row of interrupted silk mattress sutures, an intermediate row of continuous absorbable sutures, and an inner row of continuous fine absorbable sutures in the mucosa. When performing a Hofmeister-Polya anastomosis, the surgeon must take great care to overlap the suture line of the lesser curvature and the suture line of the anastomosis at the so-called fatal angle of Billroth. If proper care is taken, difficulty seldom occurs in this area. This

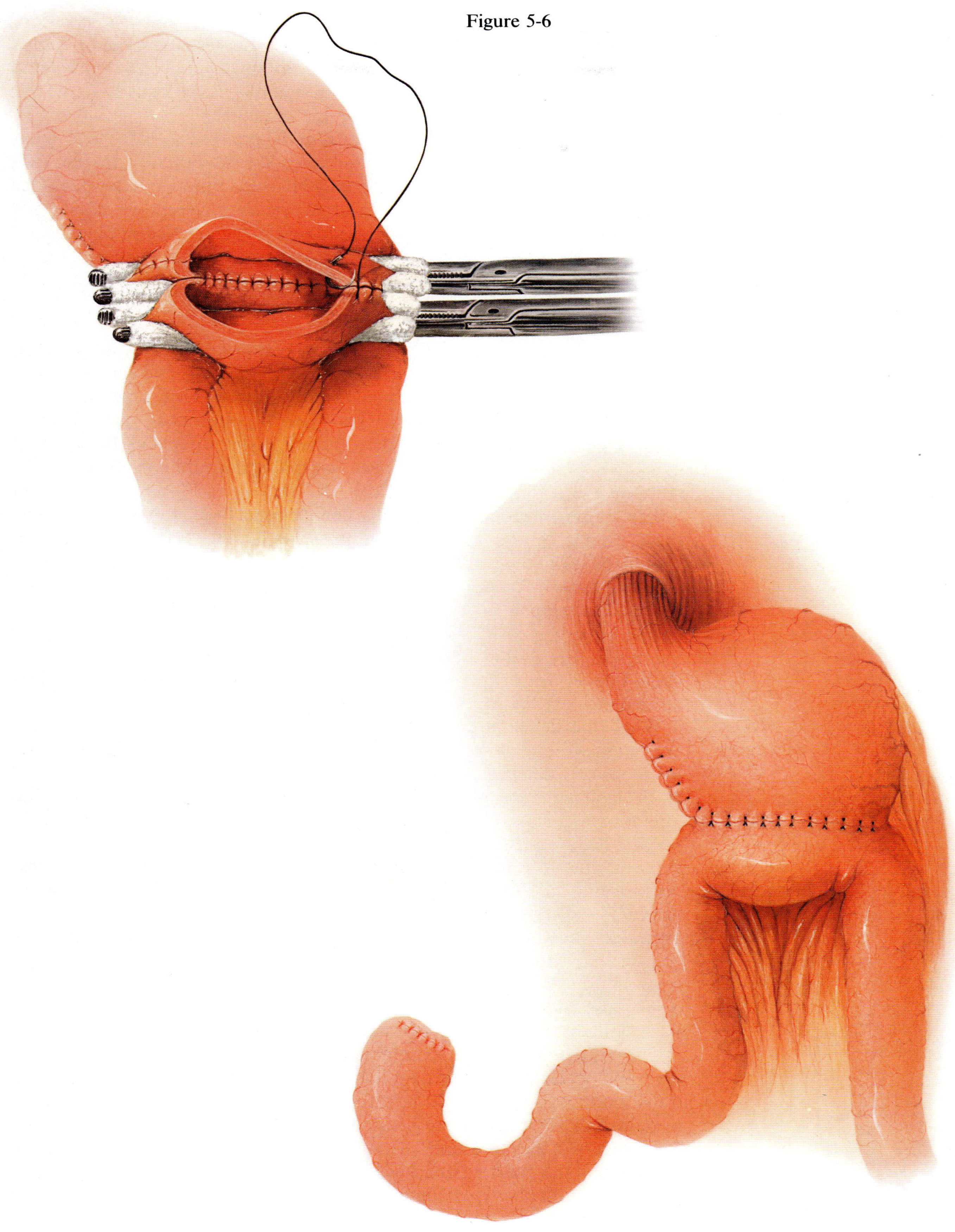

Figure 5-6

Figure 5-7

anastomosis may be accomplished in a retrocolic or an antecolic position; the type of construction is determined by whatever the surgeon deems most acceptable or desirable for the conditions at hand. The completed anastomosis (Fig. 5-7) is then adjusted so that it lies comfortably to the left of the midline without tension on the line of suture.

All free blood is carefully aspirated from the peritoneal cavity to prevent collections under the diaphragm and subsequent difficulty in the subphrenic spaces. Nasogastric suction may be used, although it has been our general policy not to use any form of gastric drainage unless conditions necessitate such a procedure. The abdomen is then closed in layers.

Total Gastrectomy

Various abdominal incisions are used for total gastrectomy, and the type to be used is determined by the habitus of the patient and the surgeon's preference. Thoracoabdominal incisions may be used, or a sternum-splitting incision may be necessary. Our general policy is to use an upper midline incision and to extend it to the left of the umbilicus for the best exposure. If more exposure is necessary, the sternum can then be split without undue difficulty.

The abdomen should be carefully and thoroughly explored to determine the presence or absence of metastatic lesions. The primary tumor also should be examined carefully for any indication of direct extension to adjacent organs. If the liver is free of any evidence of metastasis and no evidence of spread to distant lymph nodes is found, or if spread has occurred but it appears likely that the involved nodes can be removed with the lesion, then total gastrectomy may be performed. Total gastrectomy should never be performed as a palliative procedure because, under these circumstances, the morbidity and mortality rates become prohibitive.

When the decision has been made to perform total gastrectomy, the entire omentum and spleen should also be removed to eliminate all possible areas of spread to the lymph nodes (Fig. 5-1). The dissection is started at the splenic flexure of the colon and carried to the right; the entire omentum is dissected away from the colon to a point well beyond the hepatic flexure. The duodenum is then freed up carefully, as is done for a subtotal gastric resection, and all associated node-bearing tissue in this area is removed. The subpyloric nodes and superior retropancreatic nodes are removed most carefully. The duodenum is then transected (Fig. 5-2) such that a sizable part of the first portion is removed; the distal end of the transected duodenum is closed with an outer row of interrupted silk mattress sutures and two rows of atraumatic absorbable sutures, as is done for a subtotal gastrectomy. The closure is performed carefully to avoid any impingement on the lumen of the common duct.

The dissection is then continued carefully toward the left along the common hepatic artery, and all the associated node-bearing tissue is cautiously removed (Fig. 5-8). The left gastric vessels are ligated at the celiac axis, and all associated node-bearing tissue in this area is removed en bloc. The spleen is elevated and left attached to the greater curvature of the stomach by the short gastric vessels (vasa brevia), and the splenic vessels are ligated with heavy silk ligatures. Occasionally, removal of a portion of the pancreas is necessary to ensure that all of the lymph nodes in the hilus of the spleen have been eliminated. If the malignant process has extended

Figure 5-8

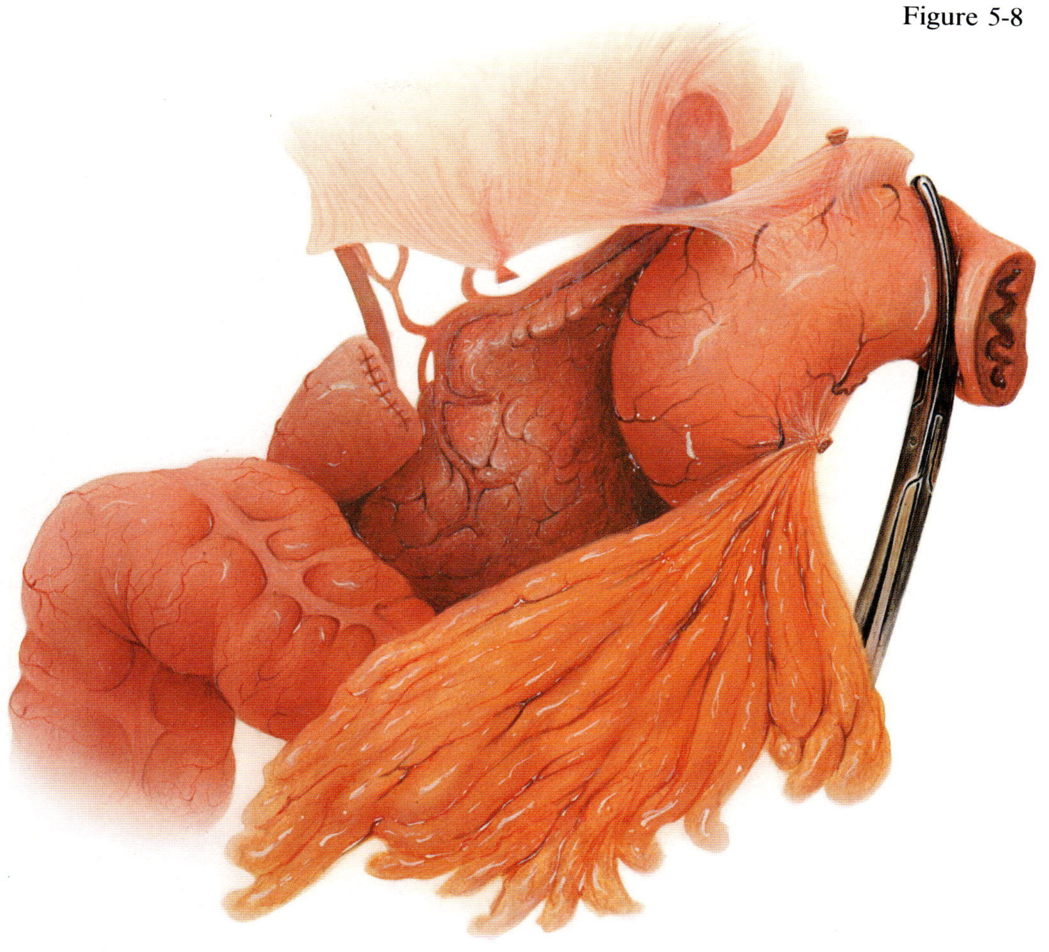

to the body and tail of the pancreas, a portion of the pancreas may have to be removed en bloc with the stomach. As mentioned previously, this step is not done routinely, but only when conditions indicate it is necessary. If a portion of the pancreas has been removed, the pancreatic duct is ligated with heavy silk material. The stump of the pancreas must be carefully oversewn with silk mattress sutures.

Figure 5-9

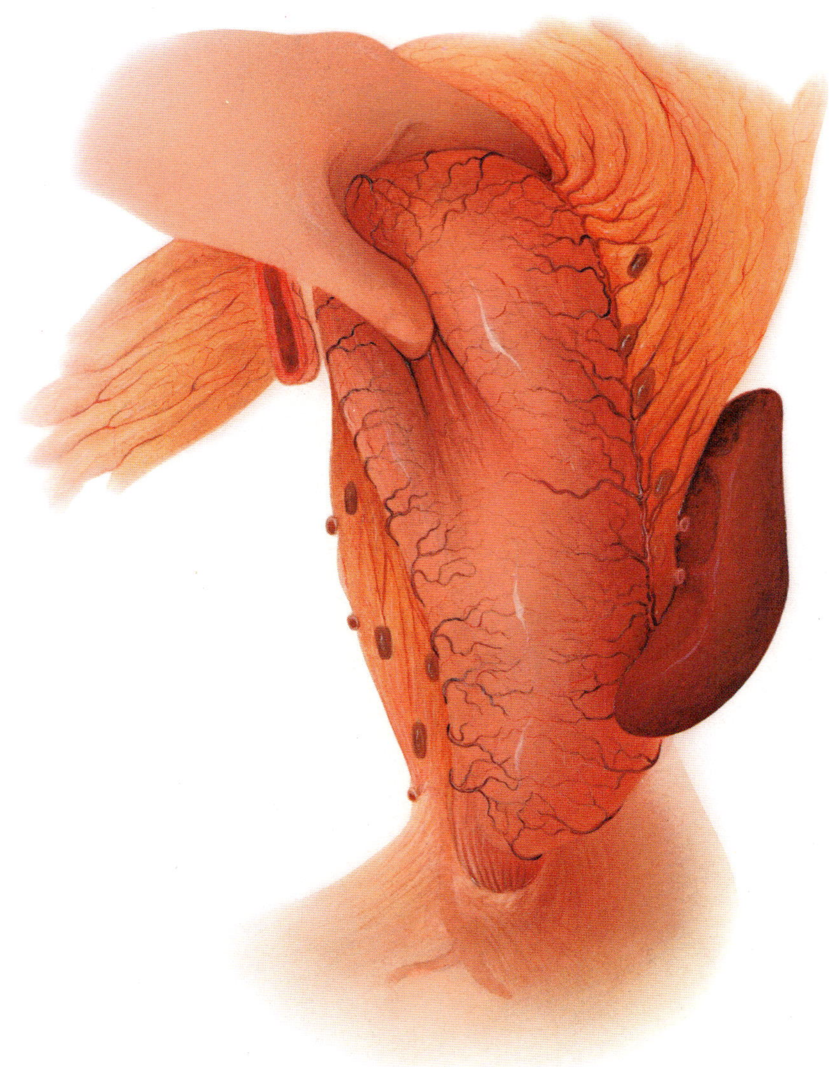

After these maneuvers have been accomplished, the stomach is free except for its attachment to the esophagus. The stomach is elevated upward and used as a retractor on itself (Fig. 5-9) to draw the esophagus into better view. To facilitate exposure of the esophagus and the esophagogastric junction, one should incise the left triangular ligament and the coronary ligament of the left lobe of the liver. This procedure frees up the left lobe of the liver laterally so that it can be retracted medially out of the operative field. The lobe is then covered with a pack and held out of the way with a Harrington or a Deaver retractor. A segment of intestine is selected from the first portion of the jejunum; it must be of adequate length so that it can be approximated to the esophagus without tension. Anastomosis of the esophagus to the jejunum is begun before the stomach is removed from the esophagus. The jejunal segment is usually best and most conveniently brought up in a retrocolic position. While making the opening in the mesocolon, the surgeon should be careful to avoid the middle colic vessels.

Figure 5-10

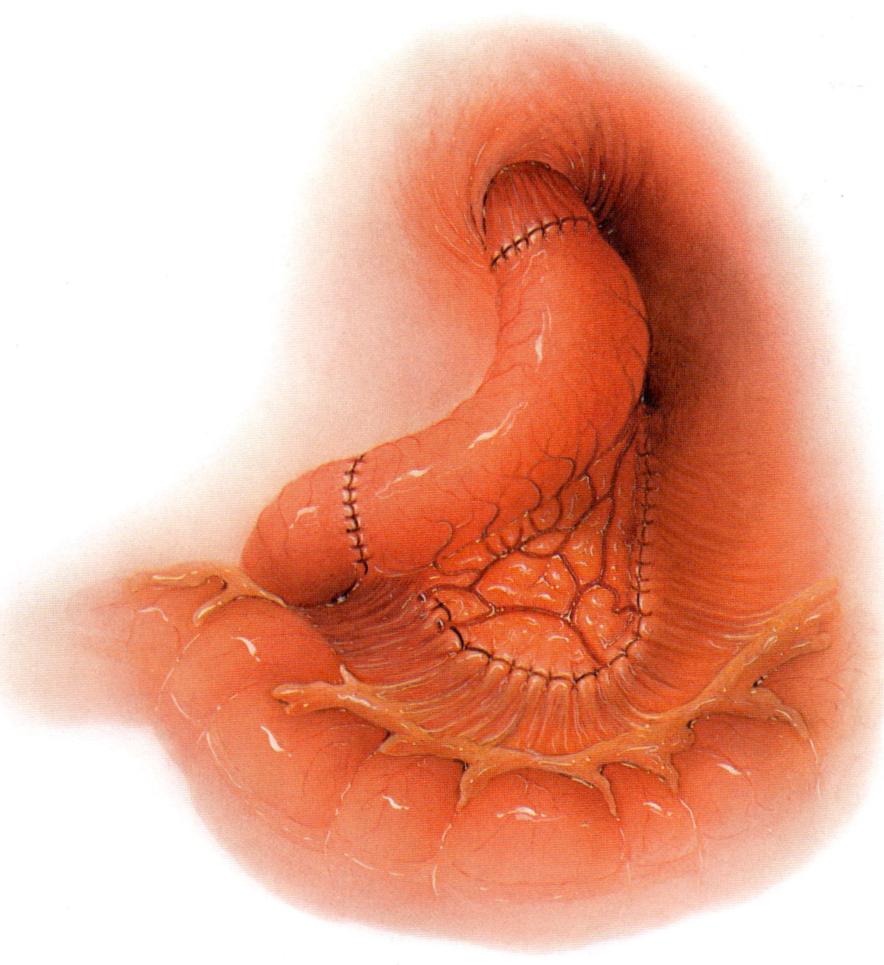

Usually, we do not use other organs as a substitute for the gastric pouch; however, an appropriate segment of jejunum (Fig. 5-10) or colon (Fig. 5-11) can be used to construct such a pouch for interposition between the esophagus and the duodenum. Such maneuvers, however, have not added to the welfare of patients nor have they, in general, contributed to their well-being.

At this point, perhaps the greatest concern, other than leakage at the anastomosis, is the prevention of reflux esophagitis from regurgitation of intestinal contents. This complication is best prevented by some form of Roux-Y anastomosis. Many variations have been applied to accomplish restoration of esophagointestinal continuity.

Figure 5-11

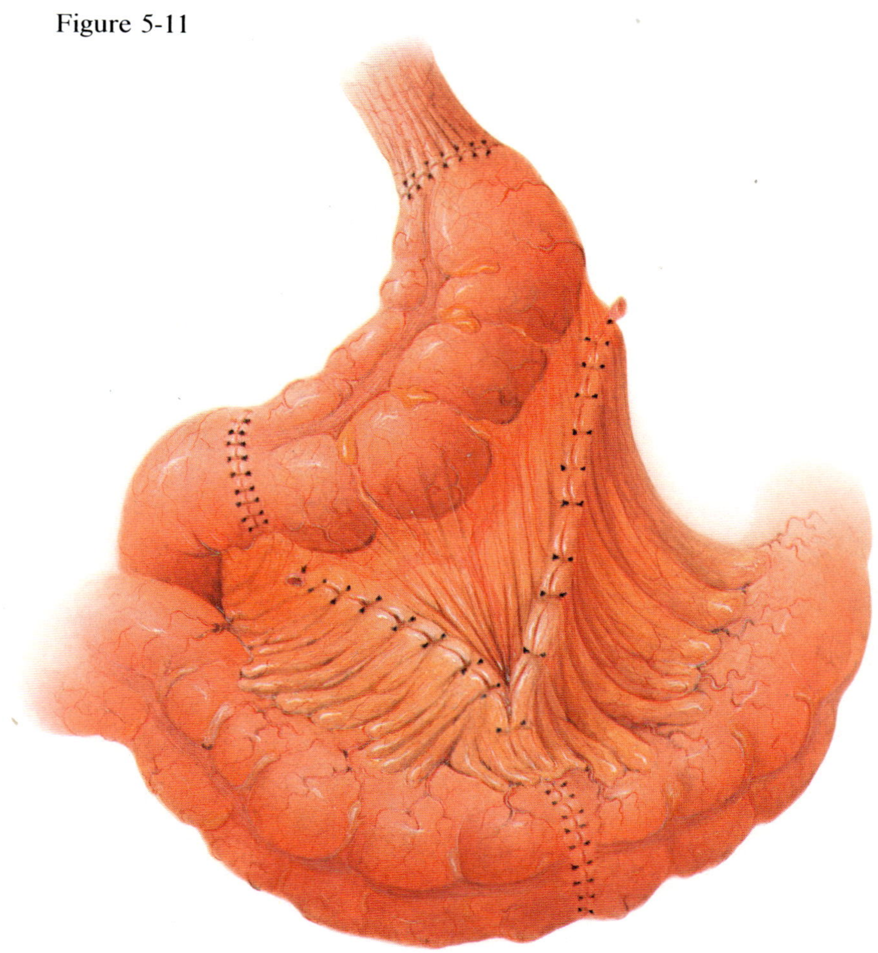

The use of a ''loop'' esophagojejunostomy was in vogue for some time, and the initial results were good. However, subsequent devastating esophagitis[7] negated an otherwise successful procedure. Further attempts to improve this procedure with the use of enteroenterostomy (Fig. 5-12) were unproductive. Extension of the enteroenterostomy (Fig. 5-13) to form a pouch did not improve the results, and esophagitis prevailed.

Our studies have shown that an end-to-side anastomosis (Fig. 5-12 and 5-13) with a loop of jejunum is associated with the lowest mortality[7] but the highest percentage of reflux esophagitis. The most successful procedure for prevention of reflux esophagitis has, in our experience, been Roux-Y. Therefore, a combination of the two approaches would have the best chance for success.

This can be best accomplished by closing the transected end of the jejunum with an outer row of nonabsorbable sutures and an inner row of absorbable sutures in the standard manner. Staple closure is also quite useful.

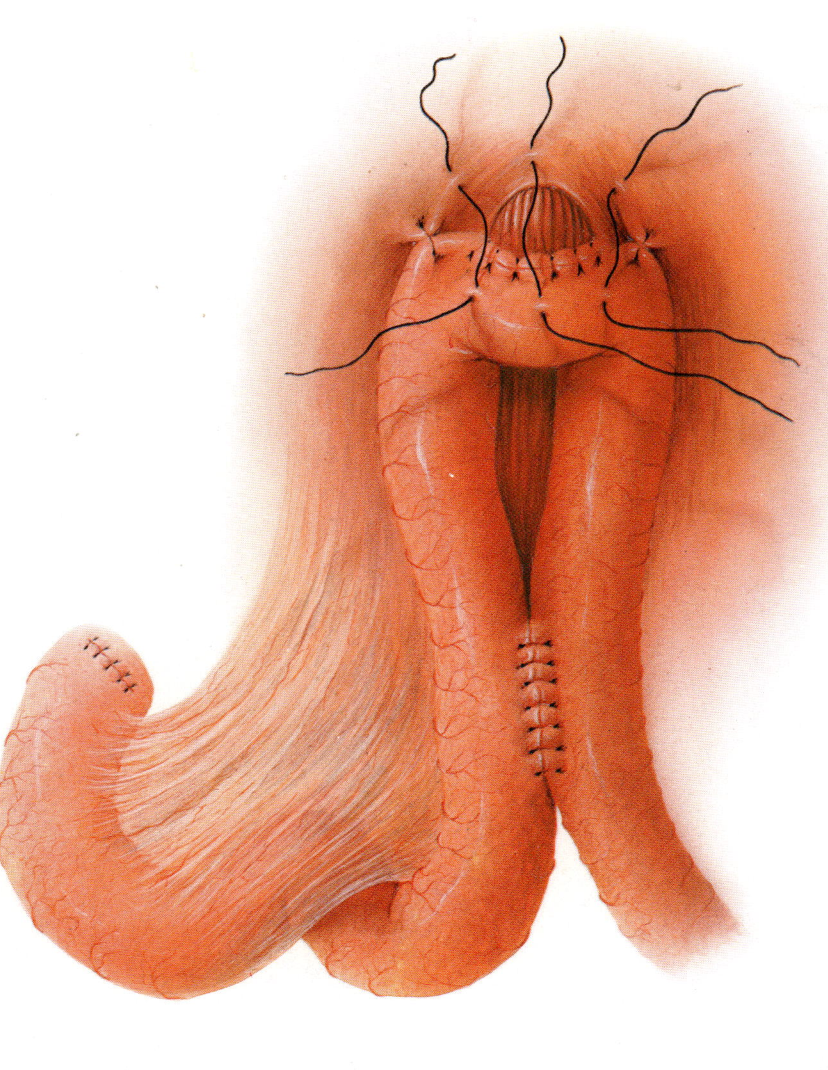

Figure 5-12

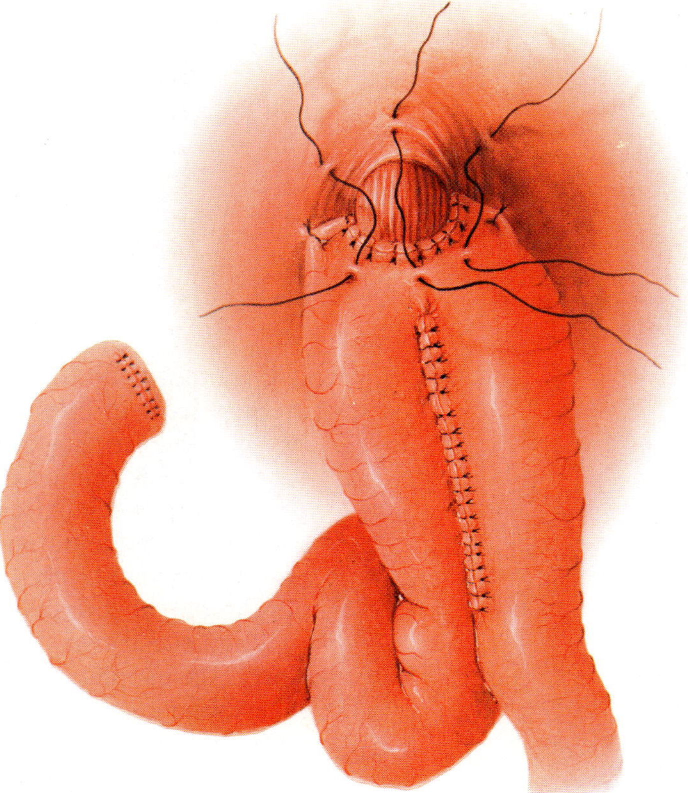

Figure 5-13

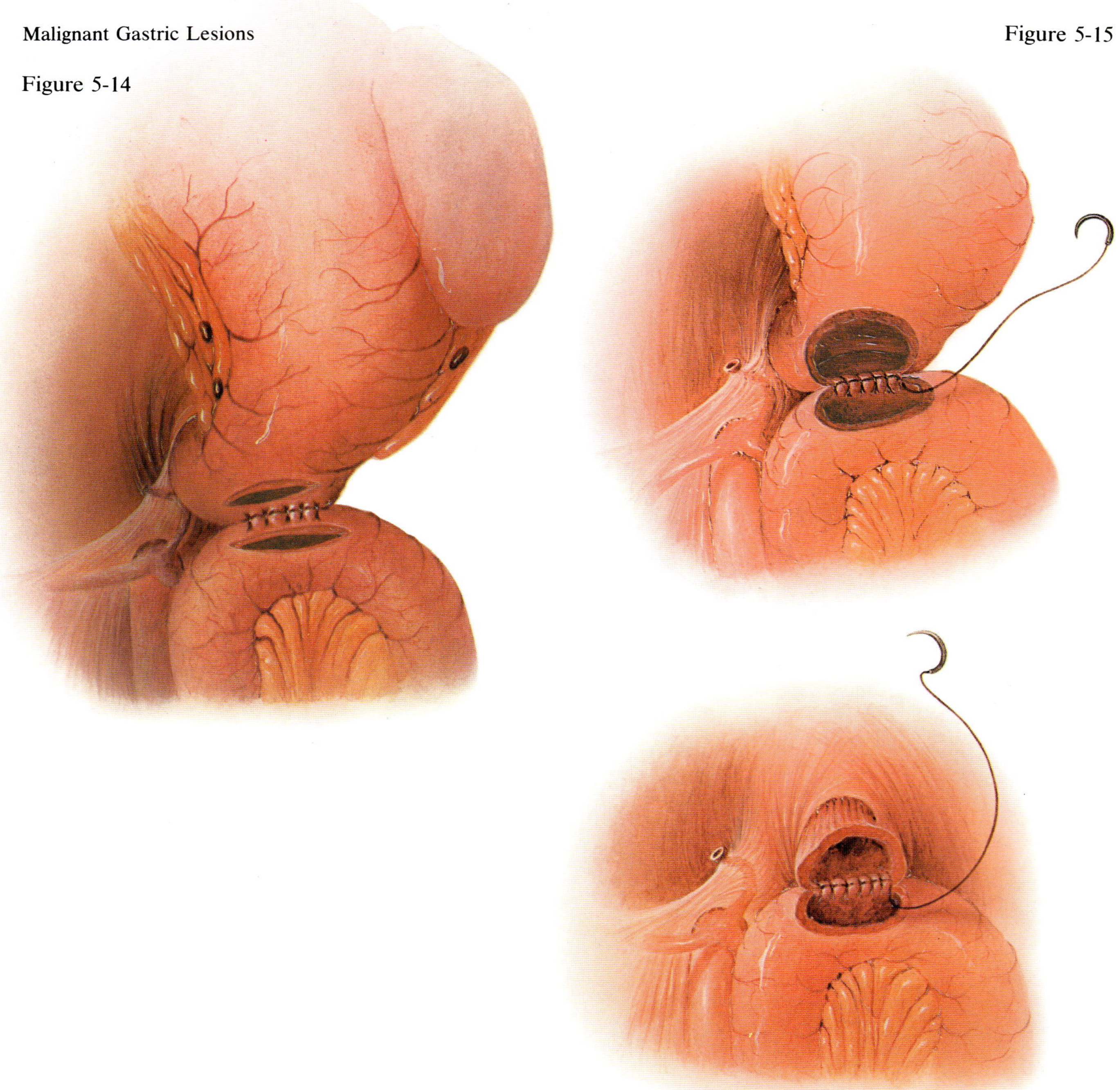

Figure 5-14

Figure 5-15

Figure 5-16

Continuity can then be accomplished in an end-to-side manner by using an outer row of interrupted nonabsorbable mattress-type sutures. Before opening the esophagus or the jejunum, these sutures must be placed transversely to accommodate for the longitudinal structure of the musculature of the esophagus. After the external row of sutures has been placed, the esophagus and jejunum are incised (Fig. 5-14) transversely on the anterior side to open into the lumen of each structure, and a mucosal layer of continuous absorbable sutures is placed.

When these two rows of sutures have been properly positioned posteriorly, the esophagus is completely transected (Fig. 5-15), and a portion of the esophagus is removed along with the stomach. The anastomosis is then completed by continuing the previously mentioned rows around onto the anterior surface of the esophagus and jejunum (Fig. 5-16); great care must be exercised in placing the sutures properly. The anastomosis is then

Figure 5-17

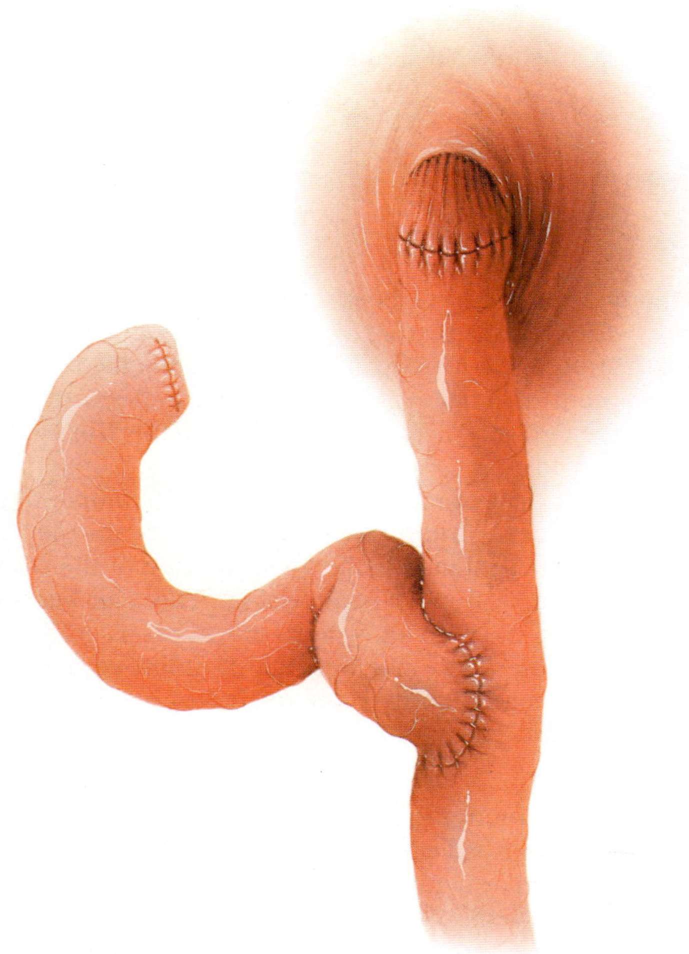

anchored to the diaphragm with interrupted nonabsorbable sutures, and a flap of diaphragmatic peritoneum is sutured down over the anastomosis to cover it and to help prevent leakage (Fig. 5-13).

The operation is then completed with an end-to-side jejunojejunostomy (Fig. 5-17) at least 30 cm below the esophagojejunostomy with an outer row of nonabsorbable sutures and an inner row of absorbable sutures.

After the anastomoses have been completed, an intestinal tube usually is passed from the nose into the jejunum through the esophagojejunostomy to a point well below the anastomosis; this tube is used for feeding purposes if a leak should develop at the anastomosis. Placement of this tube is particularly important because leakage at the esophagojejunal junction is the cause of most of the complications after total gastrectomy. As has been well known for years, the esophagus does not hold sutures well. Therefore, if a leak develops, a patient can be fed and nutrition can be maintained through the previously mentioned tube. In most such cases, healing will occur at the site of leakage, and a patient will recover satisfactorily without further surgical maneuvers. Adequate drainage of the left subphrenic space should be provided.

All free blood is swabbed from the peritoneal cavity, and a drain is inserted in the region of the duodenal stump and another in the region of the esophagojejunostomy. The abdominal closure is accomplished in a routine fashion. In the past, postoperative nourishment by mouth has been delayed longer than is necessary or advisable; however, nourishment by mouth should be started within 48 hours after operation if a patient's condition permits.

Historical Comment

Gastric Cancer

Over the years, many attempts have been made to improve the various operations that are performed to restore gastrointestinal continuity after partial or subtotal gastrectomy. Most of these operations have been devised for the management of malignant lesions; nevertheless, they have been used equally for benign gastric and duodenal problems (for example, ulcer and polyps) (Fig. 5-18).

Unfortunately, a gastric malignant lesion is sometimes inoperable because of extension to adjacent structures, seeding, or distant metastatic growths. In such cases, if the lesion is in the lower portion of the stomach with associated obstruction, a bypass is advisable. This can be accomplished in several ways (Fig. 5-19) to allow a patient to eat as comfortably as possible. These procedures may not necessarily improve a patient's longevity but they will definitely improve the quality of life.

Total Gastrectomy

Many variations for reconstruction have been used (Fig. 5-20 and 5-21). Most of these have not been as successful as hoped because of leakage or infection or reflux esophagitis or combinations thereof. In particular, operations that use a segment of the colon have been unsuccessful. In the interest of completeness, these procedures are included in the illustrations but are not necessarily recommended.

The formation of "pouches" during reconstruction after total gastrectomy is debatable. No clear-cut evidence indicates that a patient's nutritional status is improved with such procedures. We tend to discourage such operations in an effort to keep suture lines to a minimum and thereby to decrease the opportunity for leakage.

If a gastric malignant lesion is high in the stomach, is causing obstruction, and is determined to be inoperable at exploration, a feeding gastrostomy (Fig. 5-22) should be considered to avoid the use of some form of nasal gastric tube. The simplest procedure is perhaps the best. Our preference would be a simple Stamm-type gastrostomy with a "mushroom" catheter.

Gastroduodenal Anastomosis

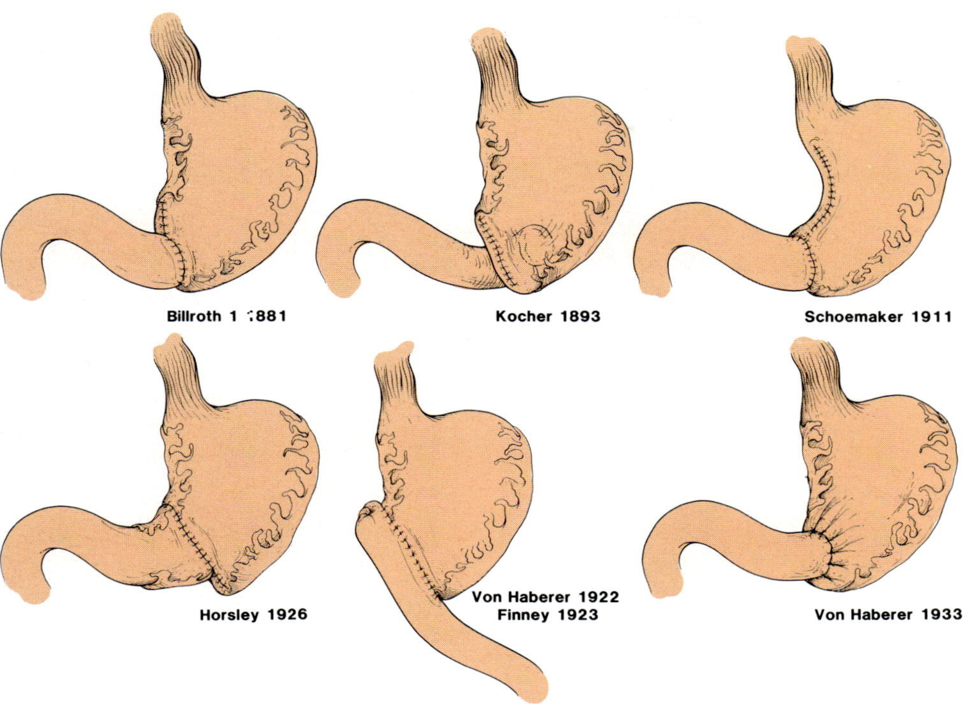

Gastrojejunal Anastomosis

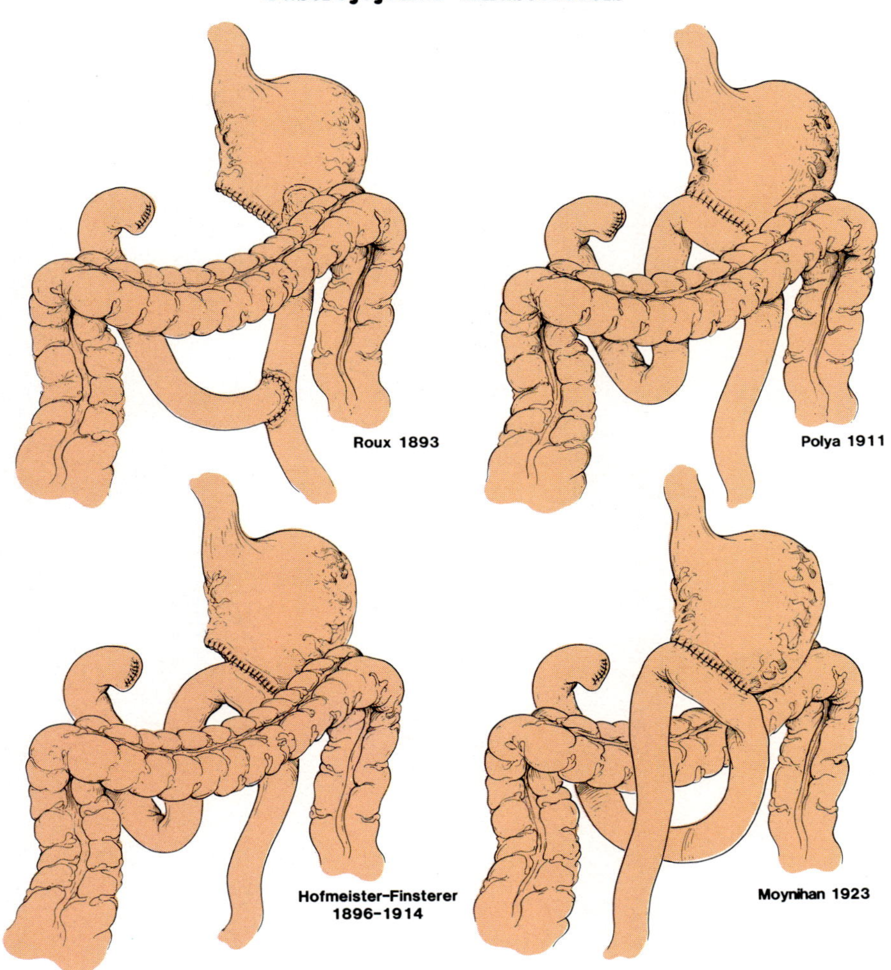

Figure 5-18

Gastrojejunostomy

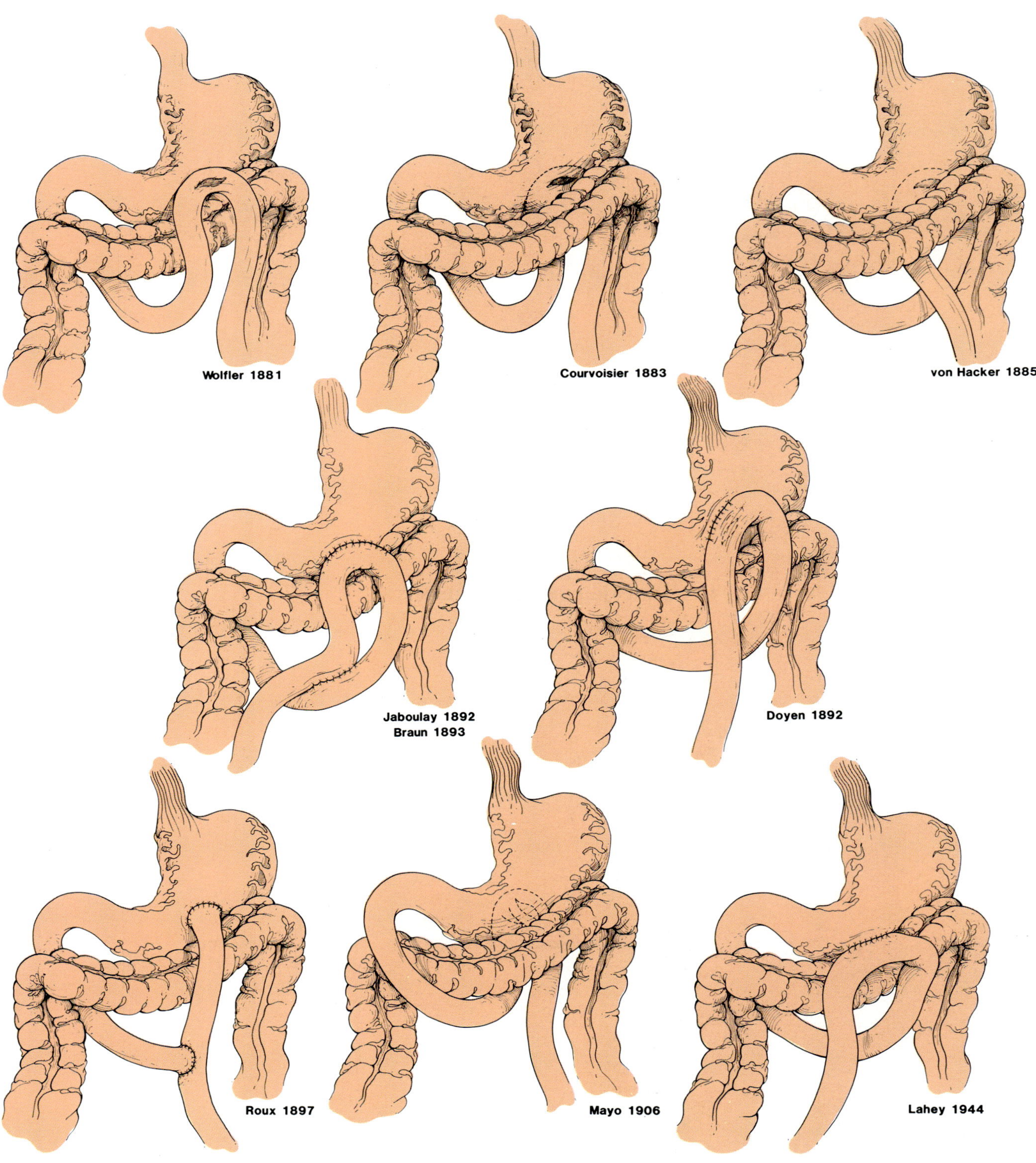

Figure 5-19

Total Gastrectomy

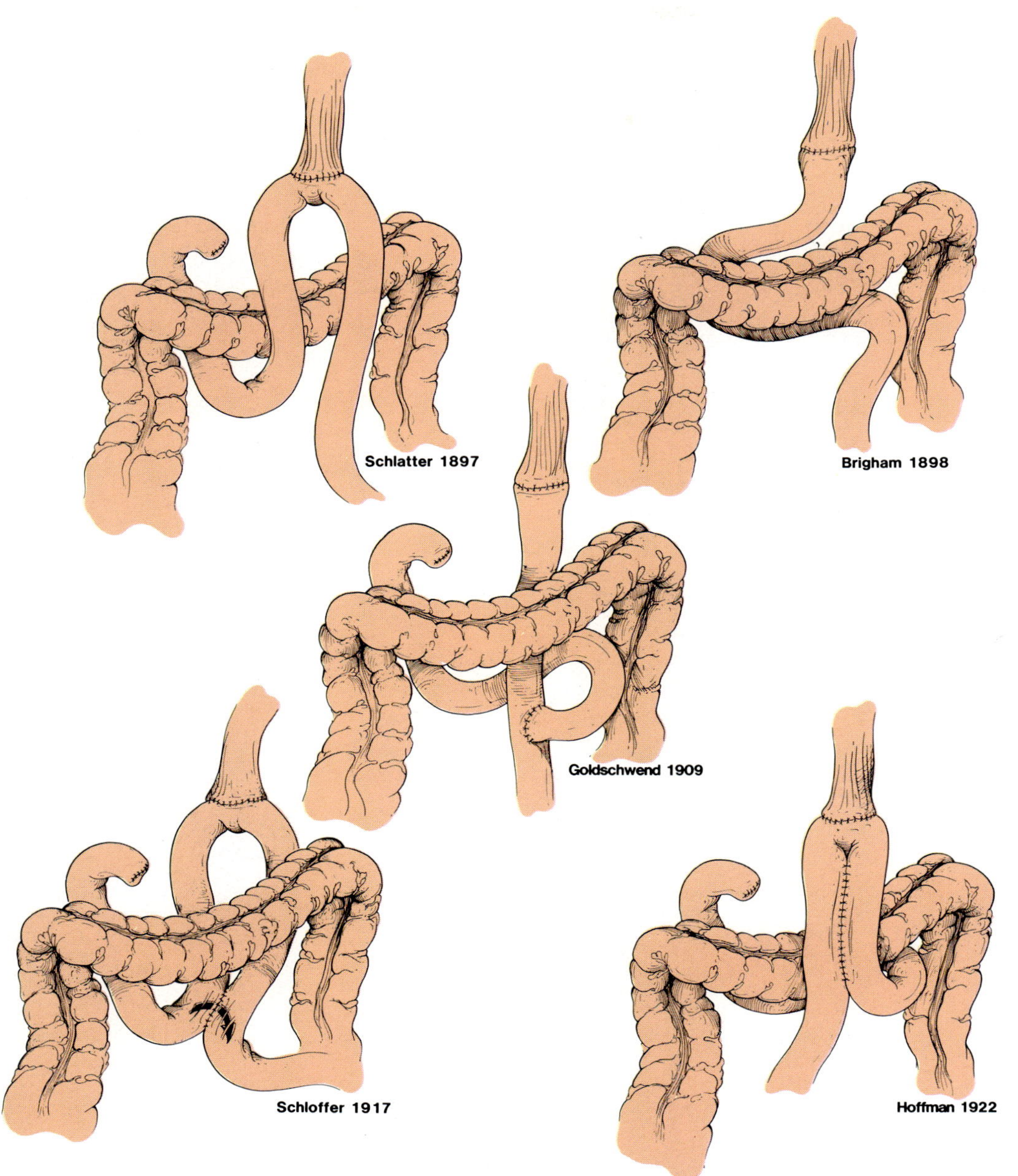

Total Gastrectomy

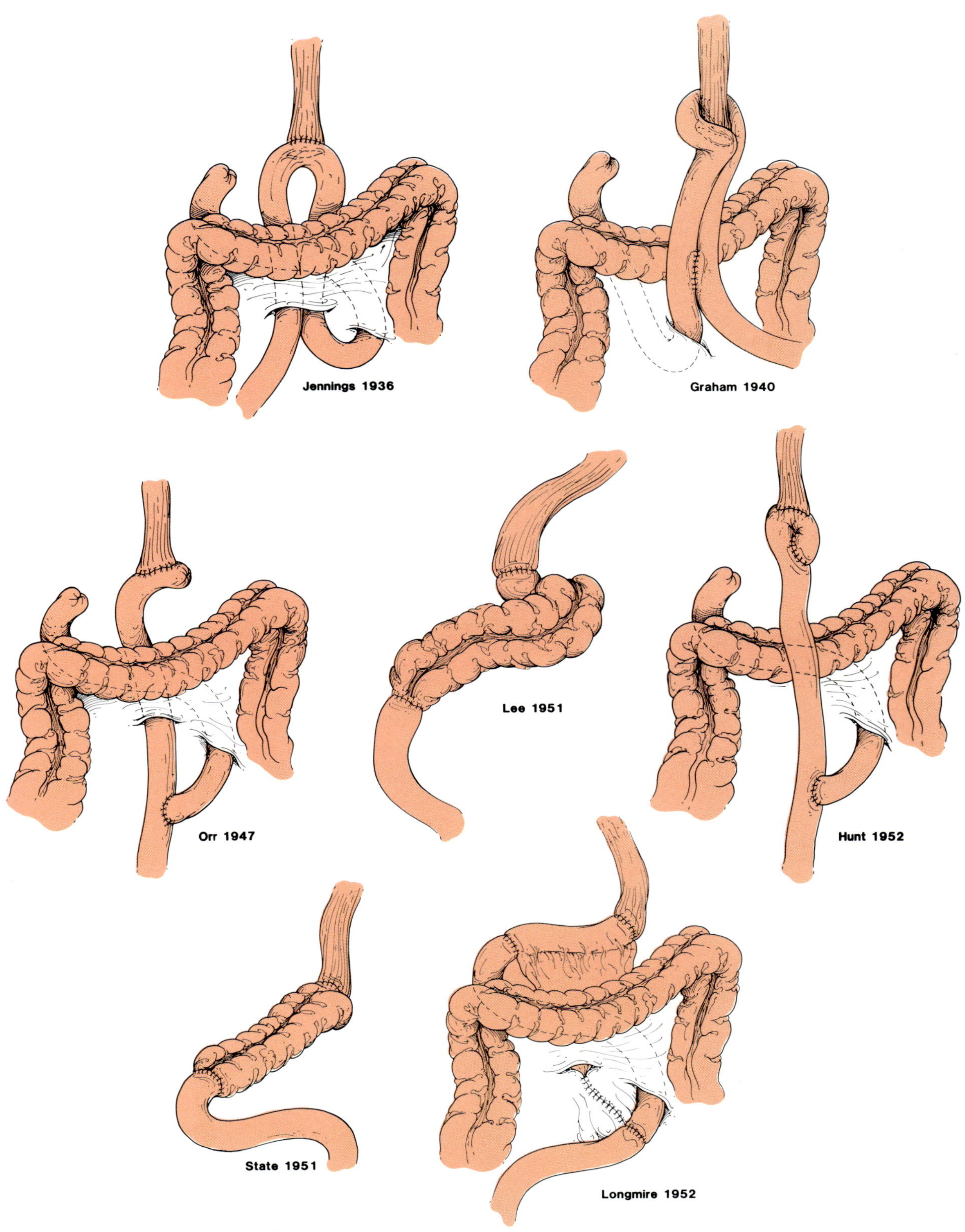

Figure 5-21

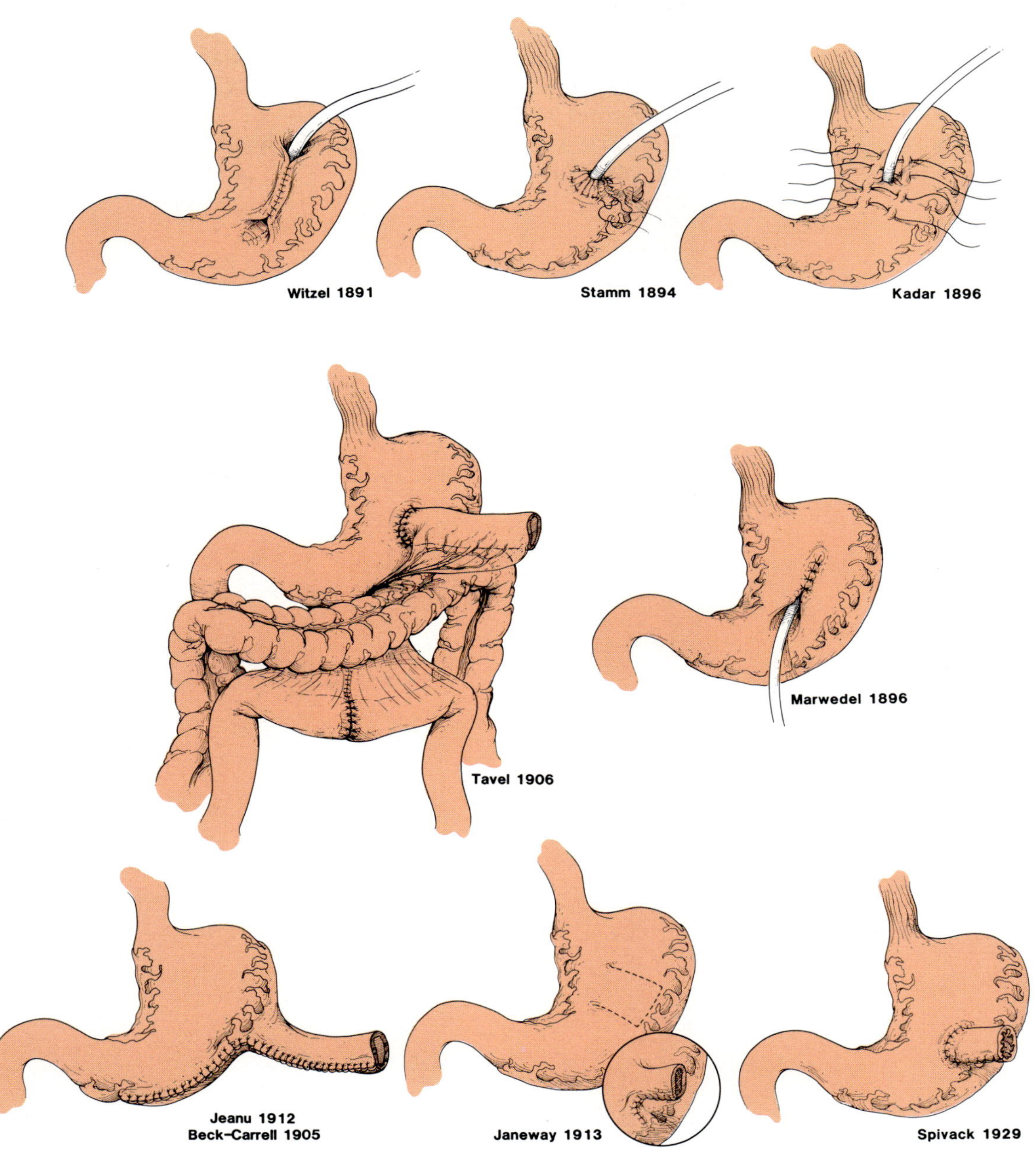

Figure 5-22

References

1. Billroth CAT (1881) Excision of a part of the human stomach; reported by JA Kasson, U.S. Minister to Austria. Month Rev M Pharm, Phila 4: 195
2. Coller FA, Kay EB, McIntyre RS (1941) Regional lymphatic metastases of carcinoma of the stomach. Arch Surg 43: 748
3. Delamere G, Poirier P, Cunéo B (1913) The lymphatics. Constable & Co., Ltd., London
4. Fly OA Jr., Waugh JM, Dockerty MB (1956) Splenic hilar nodal involvement in carcinoma of the distal part of the stomach. Cancer 9: 459

5. Larson NE, Cain JC, Bartholomew LG (1961) Prognosis of the medically treated small gastric ulcer. II. Ten-year to nineteen-year follow-up study of 391 patients. N Engl J Med 264: 330
6. ReMine WH, Dockerty MB, Priestley JT (1953) Some factors which influence prognosis in surgical treatment of gastric carcinoma. Ann Surg 138: 311
7. ReMine WH, Priestley JT (1952) Late results after total gastrectomy. Surg Gynecol Obstet 94: 519
8. Rouvière H (1938) Anatomy of the human lymphatic system. Edwards Brothers, Inc., Ann Arbor, Michigan

Index